EASY FITNESS
FOR THE RELUCTANT EXERCISER
30 DAYS TO GET STARTED AND STAY STARTED

by
Cinder Ernst

Green Ivy Publishing
1 Lincoln Centre
18W140 Butterfield Road
Suite 1500
Oakbrook Terrace IL 60181-4843
www.greenivybooks.com

Easy Fitness for the Reluctant Exerciser/Cinder Ernst
ISBN: 978-1-946775-09-2
Ebook: 978-1-946775-10-8

Acknowledgments

I have the best clients. They have helped me build the Easy Fitness system by being willing to do their fitness thing in my unconventional way. They will tell you that they are thrilled to be living their lives with strength and stamina because of Easy Fitness.

When I became a life coach in 2008, I studied at the Academy for Coaching Excellence in California with Dr. Maria Nemeth. Dr. Nemeth's books, programs, and courses taught me how to move through life with clarity, focus, ease, and grace and so I pass that onto you.

I have been developing spiritually by studying with Abraham-Hicks. I have become happy all the time and way more fun because of these teachings. These concepts fit perfectly with the message in my heart and in my book.

I want to thank my good friend Lisa for believing in me and encouraging me as we hiked the beautiful San Francisco coastline with our dogs. My loyal companion Camelot the dog keeps me sane and smiling. Thank you to Bill Young for inspiring me to find my dream and build it.

Contents

Introduction

A Small Step of Faith

I'm so happy to be writing this book for you, and I'm thrilled that you are reading it!

Welcome to your Easy Fitness journey. I know you're in the right place to receive the well-being that is here for you.

It doesn't matter what your exercise history has been, today you're making a fresh start. It doesn't matter what you look like or what you weigh, this Easy Fitness journey is not about losing weight or body shaping. Easy Fitness is simply about moving your body, getting stronger, and increasing your energy and stamina.

I appreciate that you consider yourself a reluctant exerciser. I think your reluctance is smart and appropriate. Here's why. The diet and fitness industry's message goes against your own well-being. They would have you believe that there's something wrong with you. The way they want to "fix" you is with insane fitness trends and protocols. Something inside you said *no* to that, bravo!

This book is meant to be a guide so you can find your personal path to increased strength and stamina. That is how we are defining fitness here—

having the strength and stamina to live the life you want to live. There is no shame or blame about where you are now, where you've been in the past, or what you look like.

Easy Fitness works best if you leave behind most of what you've picked up along the way about fitness. This is a new beginning; treat it as a fresh start. You'll need to have a little faith because this is going to be easier and sweeter than you are prepared for. ☺ At Easy Fitness, we call it a small step of faith instead of a leap.

Why believe me?

For starters, I've been doing and teaching fitness in this sweet, fun, and gentle way for more than twenty-five years! I've worked with hundreds of plus-size women who have gone from being reluctant exercisers to life-long movers and shakers. Through the years, I've gotten better and better at helping you find the easiest, most fun, and safest path to increased strength and stamina.

What we've got in this book are safe, simple, and streamlined systems for getting started and staying started with good-feeling exercise. There is nowhere else in the world to get this information in the way it is presented here.

I've been a personal trainer since before there was such a thing. Really, in 1988, when I pioneered the one on one training program at the San Francisco Central YMCA, there was not even a personal training certification available. Currently, I am certified as a medical exercise specialist since 1998 and an accredited life coach since 2008. These skills, coupled with my decades of experience, make me the leading expert in body friendly—no weight loss required—plus-size fitness, and these same skills will make you successful!

What you can expect in this book is a step-by-step, time-tested system to create an empowering, easy, and fun relationship with your body when it comes to fitness. You will be able to do what you said you would do about exercise consistently and without struggle.

Easy Fitness is pretty much about retraining your brain and letting your body off the hook.

The Setup

Keys

Together, we are going to tiptoe onto this new path. You can breathe a sigh of relief as you leave behind all your preconceived notions of what a fitness program should be. You will begin allowing a new foundation for your health and happiness.

This path requires a small amount of effort with a very specific focus. Everything builds from here. It's sweet and easy.

Here are two keys to your success with the Easy Fitness Systems in this book.

The first key is, nothing behind, everything in front.

You must take everything you think you know about fitness and leave it behind. All the shoulds, all the fitness prescriptions, all the trends and the advice from well-meaning others.

In place of that, you will learn to listen to your own innate body wisdom. It's there, I promise and I'll help you find it.

Nothing behind, everything in front.

The second key is, don't give a damn about what anyone else thinks.

The diet and fitness industry has nothing to do with your well-being and everything to do with advertising and profits.

Most others are brainwashed by the diet and fitness industry, and they're not ready for this leading edge Easy Fitness message. Hold what we're doing close while you are learning and beginning. Before long, you will experience you body's own confidence and feel the evidence of your enhanced energy and improved good feelings. People will begin to wonder what your secret is.

A bit about joint pain.

The exercises in this book are the same exercises I teach people in my Heal Your Knee 1-2-3 program. If you have knee pain now, you may find it diminishes over time. The same is true for back/hip and foot pain. How is that for a bonus! Easy Fitness that relieves joint pain!

How to best use this book.

Use this book as a workbook. There are times that I will ask you to do a bit of exercise in your chair . . . try it. There will be opportunities to do some sweet, mind-focusing techniques, try them too. You will find blank pages to record ahas and progress, use the pages or start a journal. Go slow. We're not in any hurry. You've got the rest of your life to figure this out. And we're gonna make it fun!

Enjoy the sweetness of this journey. Think of this book as a love song to your body.

AAA

Your Easy Fitness fresh start!

This really is a fresh start. Remember you are trying something completely different. The Easy Fitness path will look nothing like a traditional fitness path. This path will feel remarkably easy.

Remember our first key—"nothing behind, everything in front." By that I mean leave behind everything you know about exercise. Leave it behind. You are at a fitness fork in the road. You can go the way you've always gone or thought about going. Or you can try this book. This is the spot that requires a bit of faith. You've got nothing to lose and everything to gain.

How do we make Easy Fitness easy? We use simple, time-tested systems that are, you guessed it, easy to implement. Your first step on the Easy Fitness pathway begins with a system called AAA, which stands for:

1. **Alignment**

2. **Action**

3. **Appreciation**

Alignment always comes first.

I am talking about mental alignment. When I started studying with my spiritual teacher Abraham-Hicks, I learned that alignment was their most important teaching also. You can find Abraham-Hicks on YouTube or in print. Studying with Abraham-Hicks has helped me find even deeper ways to teach alignment. I'll tell you how you find your alignment in a minute. Before we do that, I want you to know why it's so important to find mental alignment first.

Without the specificity of Easy Fitness alignment, you are likely to approach this exercise thing in the usual disempowering way. The usual way is that you think something's wrong with you and so you think you should exercise. Or you think something is going to be wrong with you if you don't exercise, so you think you should exercise. Or you think you need to beat your body into changing . . . or, or, or. When you take any action from a place of shame or blame, your outcome is never really good or sustainable. That's what happens when you start out on the wrong foot. That's what happens without Easy Fitness alignment first.

Alignment first is what makes this system so different from the usual fitness stuff. The best part is that finding mental alignment is pretty easy and lovely, and it will make exercise feel pretty easy and lovely too. Easy

Fitness alignment is a specific focus that sets you solidly on the Easy Fitness path to greater mobility, energy, and fun!

Finding your alignment. Alignment is a specific focus where you put yourself in a momentary good mood. To do that, you find yourself a good-feeling thought. To do that, you will have to pay attention to how you feel emotionally.

To find alignment, you focus on a good-feeling thought. Thinking this good-feeling thought creates your momentary good mood. Easy Fitness alignment points to your good feeling now. It is purposeful. You do it on purpose. Alignment is always first.

This may take a bit of practice. Many of us have developed a tolerance for feeling lousy. For instance, you may watch the news even though it feels lousy (I know . . . you probably think you need to be informed). Then you think lousy is okay because it's familiar and everyone else does it.

You may even make your own self feel bad by beating up on yourself. If you're like most folks, you find tons of ways to prove that you don't measure up. Then you think about those things and feel bad. After that, you might even argue for your limitations. Everyone is mostly doing this. Since it's common or "normal" to treat ourselves like this, we think it's okay, yikes. Especially when it comes to exercise, traditional fitness thinking will mostly have you feeling bad about yourself. No more of that! Be easy with yourself.

How to find a good-feeling thought to create a good feeling now.

Purposefully finding a good-feeling thought takes practice. Think about someone/something you appreciate or love.

Pets are particularly good for finding that good-feeling thought because they are so easy to love. I can feel all smiley just thinking about my dog's happy head hanging out of the car window. If you don't have a pet, try a grandkid or almost any baby will do. Or a happy time, place, or circumstance. Keep it very simple. Think the thought and feel good. Try it now.

Have fun with this. Isn't it funny that we have to train ourselves to feel good? I should say retrain since we are all born knowing how to feel good. This is a focusing practice, and it's a great habit to get into. Bonus: One of the side effects of the focusing practice is that you're likely to feel good more often.

Start to notice when you are feeling good naturally, what's going through your head? The more you notice during your day when you are feeling good and what you are thinking at the time, the easier finding alignment on purpose will be. Remember, it's a practice. Feel free to make a list of things that feel good to think about and have fun thinking about them.

What if you're nowhere near a good-feeling thought?

There will be days and times when you are a bit down in the dumps or just plain grumpy. That's okay. It happens to everyone. When that's happening, find a way to soothe yourself so you can feel just a bit better. You may not be able to find a happy thought, but you can feel a little better on purpose.

To soothe yourself, move a little bit in a direction that feels a little bit better than where you are. When you acknowledge where you are and purposefully move a little bit in a better feeling direction, you will feel empowered. I learned this technique from Abraham-Hicks. They call it "forking" meaning you are at a fork in the road where you can think a thought that feels a bit better, or a bit worse. Up to you.

Here's some examples of soothing statements that work for me:

- This current feeling is temporary.
- This is not the end of the world.
- I can ride this out.
- Hang on, it'll be over soon.
- I got this.
- I'm doing just fine actually.
- I know how to make the best of things.
- I'm pretty good at finding silver linings.

- Everything is always working out for me.

If you're not feeling good (emotionally or physically), find a way to purposely soothe yourself into a little relief. Purposeful soothing for an improved feeling will raise your vibration and that is a powerful and good place to be. This is alignment too.

The most important aspect at the start is alignment. Exercise comes next.

Action.

Now let's talk about exercise, the action part of AAA. If you have resistance to the word *exercise*, notice it and soothe it. You're trying something new. Right here is a good time to check in with the first key—nothing behind, everything in front.

We are going to hook exercise to your good feeling now. We make the exercise steps very small so they don't kick up the usual fitness resistance. Let's look at more benefits to small step exercises.

All or nothing.

First, let's look at *not* a small step. This usually means all or nothing. You may know what I'm talking about. This is the usual way folks approach fitness. It's like a resolution. You know what "they" say you "should" be doing and you feel like that is the only way to go. So you decide that "this" time, you're going for it. You're gonna get to the gym three times this week or go for a walk each day at lunch or go back to water aerobics.

Fill in the blank here for yourself. Usually, this is where your reluctance kicks in. You might get it going for a bit, but it always falls away. Then you feel bad about yourself. All or nothing usually leaves you with nothing.

You're not alone. This is what happens to a majority of people when they try to start exercising. That's why I'm writing this book. To give you a different option. The small step is a big part of this system.

The power of a small step.

You get benefits from small steps that you can't get from bigger steps.

- Small steps keep you safer. You are less prone to hurting yourself when you are doing just a little bit at a time.

- Anxiety falls away when you exercise with a small step because you can absolutely do it!

- You do have the time as the small step only takes thirty seconds or a literal minute.

Here's a big secret about a small step. It's really just the next step. That is all you can do anyway—your next step. Period.

Alignment+Action.

You will be implementing a specific focus (alignment) with a small exercise (action). The combo of alignment then action is the foundation for your Easy Fitness pathway. Take your next small step in your good feeling now. And don't take that step unless you are in your good feeling now. That is the crux of this whole book. If you can do that, you will be happy and successful with fitness and life. A good-feeling thought with a friendly small step exercise . . . Easy Fitness!

The third A, appreciation is the icing on the cake.

When you appreciate yourself intentionally, you are anchoring the new Easy Fitness pathway.

When you appreciate yourself, you are also building a sweet self-accountability. Can you see what I mean about this? Good-feeling thought, the friendly small step exercise, then appreciating yourself for this accomplishment. Do you see how this habit might start to repeat itself?

Close your eyes for a moment and run through it in your head. Good-feeling thought, friendly small step, self-appreciation. Breathe.

The Easy Fitness pathway is a way for you to feel good in your body . . . right now!

AAA, relax and repeat.

The beauty of this system is that you don't need motivation because you will feel good doing what you set out to do.

You won't need to be accountable because you will be doing something that feels good. It will be an inspired no-brainer.

AAA, relax and repeat.

This is the pivot point. AAA is where you step off the traditional fitness path and step onto the Easy Fitness path. Don't look back . . . nothing behind, everything in front! And don't give a damn about what anyone else thinks.

Success Formula!

I learned this definition of success originally from my coaching mentor Dr. Maria Nemeth. Dr. Nemeth uses this way of thinking when she is teaching people how to be financially successful in her ground-breaking books *Mastering Life's Energies* and *The Energy of Money*. It was wonderful for me to study with Dr. Nemeth because she gave voice to so much of what was in my heart when it came to how I help folks feel good in their bodies.

Here is the Easy Fitness success formula:

Doing what I said I would do about exercise, consistently and without struggle.

Read the above sentence again. Can you feel the empowerment in that statement? We're going to break it down into parts so you can see how to use this formula.

"Doing what I said I would do about exercise." It's so important to decide carefully what you say you will do.

As we get started, I will recommend the specific small step exercises— that is, I will be suggesting what you say you should do. I would like you to take the suggestions and plug them into this success formula. By following the recommendations, you can get started in a safe and friendly way. As we proceed, *you* will start to determine what your best next step is.

You are your own best expert; I am your guide right now. Before long, you will be the one deciding what to do about exercise. You will be empowered to decide what is best for you, and you will have the capacity to follow through. Imagine that.

You are empowered to decide what is best for you about fitness, and you have the capacity to follow through.

Easy Fitness will feel almost effortless. Especially if you cannot worry about it. Just take one thing at a time. I tell my clients that when they get this formula down, they will never feel stuck about exercise again. Do you see that? In this program, you learn how to make smart decisions, and you have the tools and capacity (AAA) to follow through.

"Consistently and without struggle."

Pre-paving will help with Easy Fitness. My spiritual teacher Abraham-Hicks coined the term pre-paving, and it fits perfectly here with what I teach. What I mean by pre-paving is deciding a few things ahead of time. You can decide how you want to feel. You've already learned that the most important first step is alignment and how to find/look for it. You've learned that your small exercise steps will feel friendly and doable and that appreciating yourself will make this whole thing easily repeatable. AAA pre-paves your experience of Easy Fitness.

In other words, AAA pre-paves so you can exercise "consistently and without struggle." The practice of AAA brings you consistency. In the past, fitness and exercise might have felt hard in some way. You may have even liked exercise but found it hard to be consistent. That is the struggle part. There can be mental struggle; as a matter of fact, that is often the tripping point. AAA soothes that mental struggle.

I will be giving you great and friendly small step exercises with directions for making it easy so we can soothe the physical struggle. We'll be looking more at this as we proceed together. You are becoming your own expert.

Remember AAA is the foundation of your transformation. You would do well to relax into this. There's no hurry. All is well.

More pre-paving for Easy Fitness success.

In chapter 1, we will be starting with the actual doing of Easy Fitness small steps! We will spend thirty days together getting you started. To prepare for your start, I recommend that you decide on when and where you will read your page and do Easy Fitness.

Once you familiarize yourself with the small step exercise, you will need about one minute for the actual doing of it right now. As we proceed, the time will increase in one-minute increments. After thirty days, you will be up to about five minutes. I give you this detail so you can pick a time and place to try this out.

I have clients who do this with their morning coffee or tea. I have clients who do this in the bathroom, on the throne. I have clients who sit up and do it on the edge of their beds.

The easiest way to make this easy is to do it as first thing in the morning as possible. Then it's done, and you will feel empowered and successful. I find that some folks feel under pressure as the day unfolds if it's pending. You decide. There's nothing wrong. You will figure out what works best. And what feels best to you!

I have a client with a really long commute so she does AAA on her lunch break. She actually does it in the bathroom, and it works great for her. The beauty of this is that you can get it right for you . . . whatever that is. Doing what I said I would do!

One final pre-paving suggestion. Words don't teach, they just point you in a direction. Experience is a better teacher; so take a minute right now, close your eyes and imagine yourself at the time and place for your Easy Fitness practice tomorrow. Feel good about it. Reach for hopeful anticipation. Or reach for I am willing. Take a deep breath. Feel it. All is well.

Chapter 1 begins your Easy Fitness small steps! Yahoo! Here we go!

1

Start Here!

This chapter includes your first small step exercise the Tush Tilt and the first seven days on your Easy Fitness path! During these daily exercise chapters, we will be addressing both the physical aspects and the mental/emotional aspects of Easy Fitness.

You might be feeling eager and excited. You might be feeling hesitant or skeptical. No matter. We'll take it from right where you are. Say to yourself right now, "I'm doing just fine," "I am willing."

Our first super effective, strength building exercise the Tush Tilt will be done in a chair!

The Tush Tilt is the exercise we will be doing as our small step this week. The Tush Tilt is the *best* exercise to get you started building strength with ease. It works for most folks and is extremely easy to do, while giving you a great improvement.

Here are three reasons that make Tush Tilts a great choice for most folks starting on the Easy Fitness path.

- First, it's done sitting so anyone can give it a try.

- Second, it takes less than a minute so everyone has time for it.

- Those two factors relieve two big worries: I won't be able to do it physically and/or I don't have time to exercise.

Here is the problem solved, and the results you can expect from the Tush Tilt. The problem is weak butt muscles often contribute to knee pain, hip pain, back pain, and lack of mobility. The Tush Tilt (as you've probably guessed) strengthens your butt muscle. When you have more butt strength, you'll have less pain, and walking, stairs, and standing will get easier. That is a lot of result from this small step exercise.

The other problem is that butt strengthening exercises can often kick up back pain. The "tilt" in a Tush Tilt handles that by protecting your low back. The best part is that the tilt not only protects your low back, but, at the same time, it strengthens your abdominal muscles improving your core strength and stamina. When your core strength improves, your mobility and endurance increases and pain decreases. Yahoo you!

Tush Tilt Benefits:

- Increases muscle strength

- Reduces joint pain

- Improves mobility

- Easy to do

- Done sitting

Sitting posture for chair exercises.

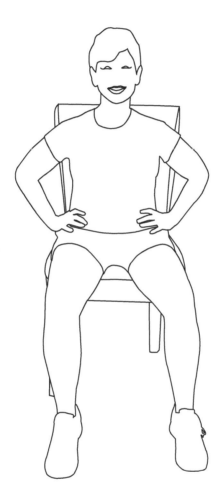

Sitting Posture

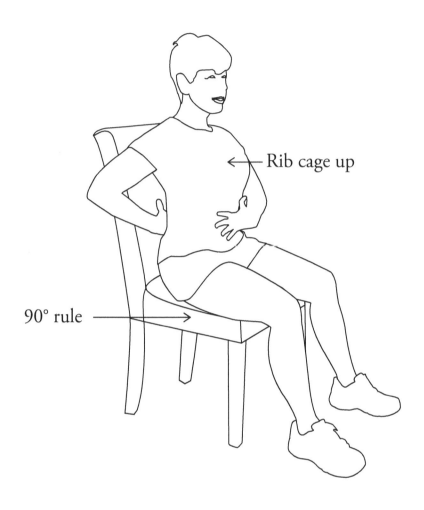

Rib cage up

90° rule

Sitting Posture

It's best to sit up as tall as you can, lift your rib cage, shoulders back and down, head . . . a natural extension of your spine. Feet flat on the floor in the ninety-degree rule, which is your ankles directly under your knees. Try the sitting posture now for practice and fun.

Go to YouTube and search for Tush Tilt or follow this link for the video tutorial: https://www.youtube.com/watch?v=DDQBv-rYhL8

Here are written directions for the Tush Tilt. Read through them. Try Easy Fitness Alignment with the movements. Stay focused and present in your body. You may not feel completely comfortable right away, but you will get there. Relax. "I am willing."

We do the tilt first. This can be tricky but don't worry, it gets easier. The tilt is actually a pelvic tilt. The idea of the tilt is to "undo" the curve in your low back while you keep your rib cage lifted.

To do that, think about pushing your navel through your spine into the back of the chair. This move will shorten your abdominal muscles momentarily, which will cause your low back muscles to lengthen and undo the curve in your low back. Try it now with Easy Fitness Alignment if you can.

To make this feel easier, try doing the navel push through with a butt squeeze. The butt squeeze helps your pelvis tilt.

Those are the two main pieces of a Tush Tilt—the tilt and the butt squeeze. To make it as safe as possible, do the tilt first and hold it, then squeeze your butt. Then release. Ta-da!

There is one more piece that will make this exercise even more valuable going forward. This piece is called the heel-butt connection. To do it, you dig your heels into the floor *gently* as you squeeze your butt. Try it now. The heel-butt connection makes going up stairs and getting up from a chair easier. More on that later. For now, all you need to do is add a small heel dig to your butt squeeze.

Tush Tilt
- Easy Fitness Alignment
- Sitting posture
- Tilt
- Heel dig butt squeeze
- Release and relax

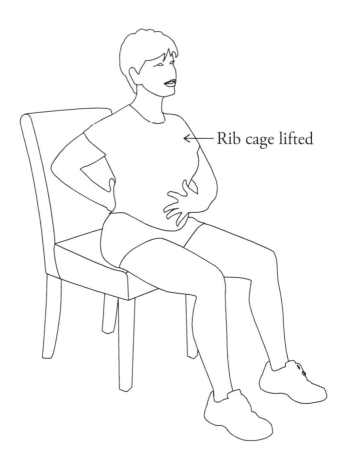

Rib cage lifted

The Tush Tilt

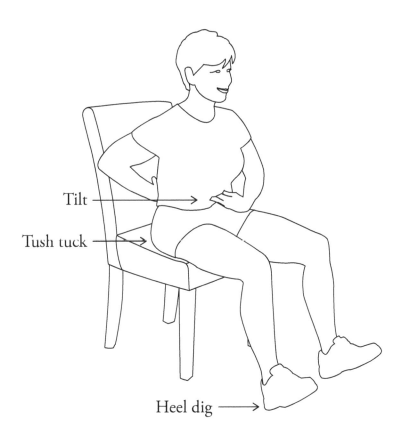

Tilt

Tush tuck

Heel dig

The Tush Tilt

Jessica's Feedback

I asked my friend Jessica May to help me with the first draft of this book. She helped me keep up with my writing by agreeing to try the system and give me feedback along the way. I wrote the page each day and sent it to Jessica. She then followed the instructions and gave me feedback. I'm including her words on many days because Jessica is brilliant, insightful, and I believe her words will be helpful to you.

I will also sprinkle in client stories and insights where they might be useful for you. Take what you like and leave the rest.

Day 1

Enough theory . . . let's go

In preparation for today, I hope you decided on a time to do this. Remember the earlier in the day, the more ease you will experience.

Here is what you do today:

1. Alignment

2. Action: 5 Tush Tilts

3. Appreciate

That's it. Breathe. Enjoy. Relax. That's all there is to it! Would it be all right with you if this were easier than you thought it might be?

Be proud of yourself for trying something lovely and different. Really, follow the instructions and see what you feel.

Remember the two keys:

Everything in front, nothing behind.

Don't give a damn about what anyone else thinks (keep this to yourself for now).

Jessica's Feedback

I enjoyed the ease of the exercise as it took only moments, creating a feeling of fulfillment and accomplishment. Similar to when I take my supplements and follow through with other commitments like keeping my appointments and caring for Buster, my roommate's dog.

I want to expose my reluctance in writing the word *exercise*. I wanted to call it activity, movement, anything but exercise. It was a literal and physical resistance and took multiple attempts to write. I found the same to be true when I was writing down when I would do the tilts. Both times, fear of failure showed up big time, as if writing this goal is a stamp of, I mean it, no turning back; I can't make mistakes; it has to be done a certain way. It was hard to stay with it, to get to "right now," and I felt the need to really stand strong, like energetically, sitting up straight, picking up my pen, redirecting my attention (hence the multiple attempts). I felt how I was being influenced by my history and found the keys to be very helpful. "Everything in front, nothing behind."

I appreciate the practice of "keeping it to myself for now." When thinking about changing anything in relationship to habits that involve my body, I have *always* shared at the beginning, talking about all the changes and plans that I would make and then would find myself out, before I was even in. You are really on to something here, Cinder. I've been wanting this kind of coaching for a long time. Bravo!

Day 2

Welcome to Day 2! Woo hoo! You're on your way.

Today:

1. Alignment

2. Action: 6 Tush Tilts

3. Appreciation

Did you do your AAA yesterday?

If yes, yay you! Maybe you noticed how nice it feels to do what you say you will do. It's just a simple lovely moment in your day. Really, it's a brave thing to walk the road less traveled and that's exactly what you're on. You are courageous!

Remember, it's a new day; nothing behind, everything in front.

(If you didn't get started yesterday, breathe, nothing's wrong, do it right now, phew. If you can't seem to find your way to AAA today, put the book away for a week and try again next week. From this point on, I'm assuming that everyone reading is doing AAA each day. Later on, we will learn how to skip a day without drama.)

Resist the urge to do more at this time. Being relaxed and easy about this is your new Easy Fitness path.

Remember that sometimes it might be tricky to think that good-feeling thought if you are not in the vicinity of feeling good. Notice where you are, how you are feeling right now. It's all right no matter where you are. Find a way to soothe yourself.

You don't have to be perfect (even though you are). Some days will be harder than others. So it stands to reason that some days will be easier.

You can figure this out as you go. Just find the best feeling thought from where you are right now. We'll be doing it again tomorrow so there's always another chance.

Day 3

1. Alignment

2. Action: Try 7 Tush Tilts today if it feels right to you, or stick to 5 or 6 if that feels right.

3. Appreciation: Yay you! Every little bit counts

How're you doing with the alignment piece? The partnering of a good-feeling thought with your small sweet exercise is the foundation for your success with the Easy Fitness system.

The feeling of alignment (thinking a good-feeling thought) first is so important at this time. It's like you are laying new pipes, through which, your strength and mobility will come through. You've got to have the pipes.

Some folks find the alignment piece harder than the actual exercise piece when we begin. Don't worry if that's happening to you, you're not alone. We have become tolerant of feeling negative. We worry, we criticize, we victimize ourselves and others, we watch the news, we argue on Facebook, we are influenced in so many lousy feeling ways. It would not surprise me that making a habit of thinking a good-feeling thought takes some effort when you are beginning.

Remember, I'm not asking you to think positively, only that the thought you think feels good. I love seeing my dog's head out the window in my side-view mirror. I feel so happy. I think that thought over and over again. That's the kind of thought you're looking for here. Something sweet and simple.

Here are some points to consider or to write about.

- What are you noticing about alignment?

- What are you feeling in your body at AAA time?

- What are you feeling in your body during the rest of your day?

Jessica's Feedback

I was distracted and felt myself negotiating my AAA time this morning, felt like it could be put off until later. I found myself renegotiating my exercise time so that I could do other things. Renegotiating exercise is an old habit. Because my plan is to exercise, take my supplements and journal, I realized that I needed to get some water for my supplements to support doing my thing. This is a valuable realization in preparation. I am noticing that accomplishing AAA is motivating me in other ways including connecting with friends, laughing at Buster's silliness and overall just saying "yes" a bit more often. I also feel lighter both physically and mentally.

Starting exercise takes me a minute to fully align with my breath and posture. So far, I've had to "practice" first to get the tilt technique down while breathing. I find myself conscious of the pace, so when I felt rushed, I slowed down; that definitely added the feeling of intention.

Day 4

It Just Feels Right

Easy Fitness is a system. It's repeatable. It's proven to work. Remember, we have twenty-six more days together so there's no need to be perfect at any of this at this time. Just relax into the system.

Part of the system is you figuring out what feels right to you. In the beginning, my guidance about choosing an exercise is important because it will keep you safe and help you not get stuck. As we go along, you will want to check in with your body about what we're doing and how it feels. That is why we increase a little bit at a time. So you can learn the subtle voice and opinion of your body.

Each day, we are adding one Tush Tilt . . . if it feels okay to you to do that. It should always feel friendly. Your body should feel happy to cooperate. If adding an additional Tush Tilt feels uncomfortable, don't do it. Wait till it feels friendly and then do it.

After you are in alignment and doing your exercise, see if your body is saying anything. It might feel relieved to be moving; it might just feel happy and relaxed and cooperative; it might not be saying or feeling anything that you can hear just yet. No worries. Just be present when you're squeezing and see what you see.

So if it feels friendly and doable…

1. Alignment

2. Action: 8 Tush Tilts

3. Appreciation

Jessica's Feedback

This morning, as I looked at my day, it became like a checklist (take supplements "check," do Tush Tilts "check"). I used my breath meditation practice to ground me and really focus during my exercise and before I knew it, I had done eight tilts.

With my brain being in alignment, the chatter stops, and I'm able to focus on and appreciate the exercise without any attachment to results.

I feel an excitement, one that I think I have to monitor. It's that "well, if I can do this, then more is better" excitement. It's funny. I recognized my own excitement by remembering the training that I practice with Buster. When he is excited, I manage it with calm assertive energy; what a perfect way to align with my Easy Fitness system.

Day 5

Appreciation!

1. Alignment

2. Action: 9 Tush Tilts if you want to

3. Appreciation

Take a moment and really appreciate yourself right now . . . for finding your way, for keeping a promise, for caring about yourself. Appreciation is a habit of thought similar to alignment being a habit of thought. In the Easy Fitness system, we ask that you appreciate every accomplishment, no matter how small. This is part of why the small step is so important, so you can develop your appreciation muscle.

I want to make a distinction here about appreciation and gratitude. Fill in the blanks here and notice the difference:

Today, I am grateful for _____

Today, I appreciate _____

I like appreciation because it has an active, present quality. To appreciate is a verb. When I look for and find things to appreciate, I feel alive and empowered. To be grateful describes a state of being. This is also lovely. I have noticed that I often use gratitude in response to something else . . . when I need to be reminded that I am grateful.

AAA trumps accountability and motivation!

Enjoy your appreciation muscle. This appreciation piece is how you develop your own self-accountability. But it's different from what most folks mean when they speak of accountability. When you use AAA, you don't need accountability. Appreciation sets you up to feel good about what you are doing. When you feel good about what you are doing, it's easy to do it again. It's that simple.

You don't need motivation when you feel good about what you are doing either. Motivation is what people do when they are taking an action, because they fear what might happen if they don't take that action. Easy Fitness is about feeling good bringing about more feeling good. When you use AAA, you don't need motivation.

A few notes from Jessica:

I am grateful for today's alignment.

I appreciate my new exercise tools.

It's funny, I was thinking that tomorrow is Saturday, a day off. That thought was quickly followed by the realization of my daily commitment—*every day*! Today, I choose to appreciate the feeling that I get from keeping my promise, the feeling of accomplishment and self-determination.

Day 6

I Am Willing!

You've done five days in a row of exercising! Today will be the sixth!

1. Alignment

2. Action: 10 Tush Tilts

3. Appreciation: Yahoo you!

Are you willing to make it ten Tush Tilts today? Does it feel like the right thing to you? There is no pressure to be at ten Tush Tilts today. Only do that if it's right for you. I've tried to pace this so it serves most, but that doesn't mean it serves everyone. You decide. Part of the beauty of this approach is that you learn to do what's right for you.

You have been willing to try something new. Give yourself a pat on the back. Being willing is one of your greatest strengths. Here is more wisdom I learned from Dr. Nemeth:

- You can be willing to do what you don't want to do.

- You can be willing to do what you're scared of doing.

- You can be willing to do something you don't even know how to do.

- Try writing "I am willing" on a post it and gaze at it.

I hope this system is feeling friendly to you. And maybe expansive. Like you're on to something here. You are building a new pathway. Maybe it feels exciting. Maybe you feel eager. Maybe you are simply willing to let it unfold. Bravo.

How is your body feeling?

What are you noticing?

Tomorrow, we will talk about taking a day off and you can decide if that's right for you.

Jessica's Feedback

I am willing!

Until I read your affirmation of completing six days of exercise, I had not put it all together. Part of being willing is to be prepared. Today, I noticed that by not having my water jug filled and an ink pen to journal, I became distracted by playing computer games and watching videos. Being willing helped me to get prepared in an unprepared, unaligned state of mind.

I notice that my sciatica is responding positively to my regular exercise. I also noticed that the tilts are reminding me to use my Tush muscles when getting to a standing position throughout the day. I noticed that the gradual increase helps me to remain present and in appreciation of completing my exercises while challenging my mental alignment at the same time.

Day 7

A Day of Rest

Today is the last day of our first week. Consider taking a rest day today. Tomorrow begins chapter 2 and our second week. We will be learning two upper body exercises, a hamstring stretch and some more Easy Fitness guidelines.

Momentum. You have exercised in this sweet and friendly way for six days. I encourage a daily practice so you can build some momentum on your Easy Fitness path. You might be feeling like AAA Tush Tilts is pretty easy, yay.

Are you feeling relief or maybe happy that you are taking care of yourself in a new and lovely way? You might be enjoying the feeling of accomplishment. You may be excited about the possibilities. If you are noticing some struggle, don't worry. That will ease up along the way. I'll give you some tips about that tomorrow.

Today, let's talk about taking a day off. Taking a day off is great practice for starting back up. Take today off, start back up tomorrow. The Easy Fitness system is designed to make starting and stopping easy. Everyone gets sidelined, sidetracked, or offtracked sometimes; that means you're human. Easy Fitness offers a way to get back on track without drama. No drama is the key to getting back to your practice. So take today off and start back up tomorrow. It's good practice.

No matter where you are in your exercise practice, Easy Fitness has your "get back on track" plan. Here's how it works today and in the foreseeable future. AAA + Tush Tilts is your key to getting back on track when you need to. Just tuck this away and know that anytime in the future when you do AAA + Tush Tilts, you are officially in that moment on the Easy Fitness pathway and all is well!

So today, if you want, let's practice the skill of getting back on track with no drama.

Take today off.

Get back on tomorrow.

See how that feels.

Yahoo you!

Jessica's Feedback

I am really enjoying the feeling of accomplishing my exercise goals. I am also happy that by exercising, I am able to accomplish other tasks throughout the day. I appreciate the tools for getting back on track. Though my struggle today was more about preparedness, using alignment and the simple tilts is a good redirection on those harder days. Again aligning my mind is the key.

2

Hamstrings, Swimmers, and Our Second Week

Week 2!

You're on a roll. Can you feel it? You may have experienced both ease and struggle this past week. That just means you're human. Any combination of ease and struggle is fine. We will visit the ease and struggle topic throughout the book.

Struggle. You may notice that you are getting better at handling struggle because you are getting better at AAA. You might get to the point where struggle is *not* a big deal, it's just normal. You simply find a way to soothe it and move on.

Ease. When you are experiencing ease, I suggest that you milk it a little. Take a moment and acknowledge what the ease feels like and enjoy it. Bask in it. Also, take credit for the ease. You are specifically taking actions (AAA) that help to create ease, and it's working. Do you feel empowered knowing you have control over how you are feeling?

Looking ahead this week.

This week, I'm suggesting you add the all-powerful Hamstring Stretch.

We will also look at adding an upper body exercise combo including Shoulder Rolls and an exercise called a Swimmer. I will include complete instructions here and abbreviated instructions on the day we add on.

The nature of adding on will mean that you have to be ready. Ready to add a minute. Ready for a bit more activity. Ready to give it a try and see if it's the right thing for you. Remember, go easy on yourself. You can take as long as you want to move through Easy Fitness. The page a day is only a suggestion. You know you better than anyone!

Easy Fitness means that you increase in a friendly feeling, small step way. Once you learn the movement, the Hamstring Stretch will add about one minute (or less) to your exercise routine. The Swimmer combo will also add less than a minute.

Meet Your Hamstrings

The hamstring muscle is the back of your thigh. It goes from behind your knee up to your pelvic bowl or hip area. Think under your butt. When this muscle is too tight, it can cause knee, back, hip, and foot pain. Yikes! Stretching this muscle sometimes helps resolve those pain issues. Keeping this muscle flexible can also prevent all those joints from becoming painful. Those are some cool reasons to stretch your hamstrings, don't you think? I get excited by these little exercise steps that have such great potential for good.

Bonus: Calf stretching included! Your calf muscle starts behind your knee and connects at your ankle. Tight calf muscles contribute to knee and foot pain, and it can sometimes lead to plantar fasciitis. If your calf muscles are tight (and it's pretty common that they are), you will feel them stretch during the hamstring stretch positions. This is perfectly fine. Some people only feel the hamstring stretch in their calves until they loosen up a bit, so that's fine too. Whatever is tightest will get the chance to stretch first. Be easy about this. Pay attention.

Some general stretching guidelines.

- Be gentle. The stretch should feel small or medium. Never big. If you stretch too hard, your body will sometimes react by tightening up.

- Hold in a comfortable place for fifteen to thirty seconds.

- The hamstring stretch goes really well right after the Tush Tilts because the area gets a little warmed up and then the muscle stretches easily.

Here are some positional options for stretching your hamstrings with a calf stretch bonus:

My favorite, the Famous Flop Over. Stand facing your bed, legs pretty straight, front of thighs touching the edge. Bend forward from the waist and let your upper body rest on the bed. You may feel this stretch from your back down to your heels. Remember gentle, hold for fifteen to thirty seconds.

Alternative Flop Over. You can do this almost anywhere. Stand facing your chair or toilet. Legs straight, bend from the waist, and put your hands on the seat. If you need more stretch, you can put your forearms on the seat. You can also do it by your desk, table, or counter. Legs pretty straight, then bend at the waist and support yourself on the surface in front of you. Play with this because stretching your hamstrings is fun to do almost anywhere.

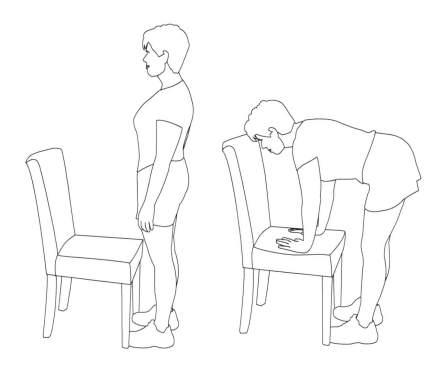

The Flop Over

Seated Hamstring Stretch. Sit in good posture. Straighten your right leg keeping your heel on the floor. That alone may get you the stretch. If not, stick your butt out a bit and see how that feels. You can also flex your foot which may get you a calf stretch too, which is a good idea. Then try the other leg. Often your legs will feel this differently from side to side.

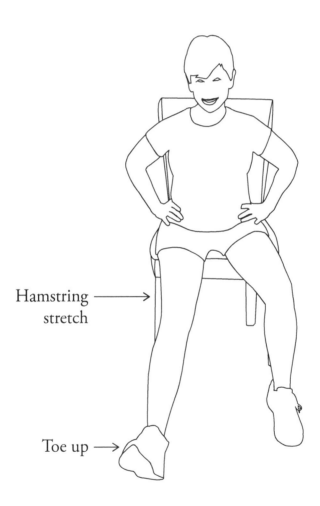

Seated Hamstring

Remember Your Calf Muscle

Your calf muscle is the back of the lower leg. Sometimes if your calves are pretty tight, that is where you will feel the hamstring stretch first and that's just fine. When your calves loosen up a bit, then your hamstrings will be more stretchable.

Try these positions and pick the one that works best for you and your body. Hold for fifteen to thirty seconds.

The Swimmer

The Swimmer is an upper body exercise. As with all our Easy Fitness small steps, this one packs in a ton of benefits. Shoulder Rolls are the perfect warm-up for Swimmers so they work well as a combo.

First, here's the problem that Swimmers help solve—the slump hump in your back. You know how as we get older posture changes often give you a hump at the top of your back? Neck, back, and shoulder pain often come with the hump. The Swimmer can improve or prevent the slump hump. "Un-slumping" when you notice you're slumping is also highly recommended!

The hump comes from our natural tendency while sitting, driving, reading and/or computing to let ourselves slump forward. Your shoulders round forward and your head follows suit, and you can develop a slump hump. The muscles in your chest and front shoulders shorten, and the posture muscles in your back loosen and get weak. The Swimmer loosens the front and strengthens the back of your shoulders, allowing you to have a more upright posture.

Bonus: The Swimmer is a self-correcting exercise for upper back and neck pain!

Modifications. The Swimmer, done with full range of motion, will have you put one arm at a time straight over head as if you were raising your hand in class saying "pick me." Here are some modifications if you have neck or shoulder pain that limits your pain-free range of motion. None of this should hurt, ever. If one or both arms will not go overhead, you can stop at chest height or shoulder height. Find your way by noticing where the discomfort begins and then stopping before that. Our rule about this: No pain, no pain. If you can't find any pain-free range of motion with this exercise, then stick to the shoulder rolls for a few weeks and try again later. Remember, we're in no hurry. All is well; we're wanting this to be just right for you.

Shoulder Roll instructions. You can roll forward and/or back. Go easy. Be deliberate going forward, up, back and around, or the reverse.

Swimmer instructions. Start by doing it in a chair. Sit on the edge of your chair if you have a chair with arms so your hands can hang down. Good sitting posture is ninety-degree leg position with your ankles under your knees, rib cage lifted, and your head being a natural extension of your spine.

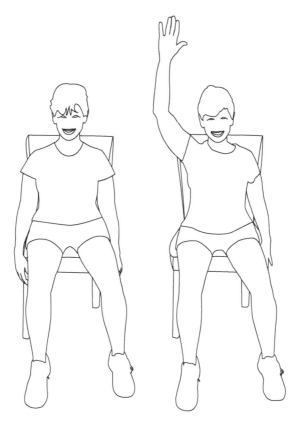

The Swimmer

- Now raise your right hand in the air as if you wanted to be called on by the teacher.

- Modification: You can have your palm facing front. Or you can have your palm facing in. One position may feel friendlier than the other. Try and see. Remember only lift your arm to a height that is comfortable.

- When you raised your hand, you probably just put it up from your side. We want something a bit different.

- We want your arms to move as if they were straight arm levers moving up and down in front of your body. The swimming motion comes as one is going up, one is coming down. Your straight arms should pass each other at about chest height and reach their up/down destinations at the same time.

- Pause with one hand up in the air and one hand down at your side, then switch the positions. Move deliberately and smoothly.

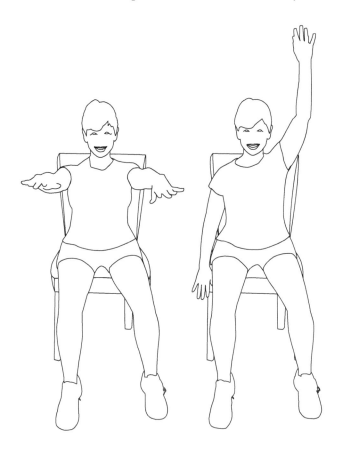

The Swimmer

Here's how the muscles are working. At the top of the motion, the back of your shoulder is getting stronger at the same time as the front of that shoulder is mobilized or stretching. This is a basic anti-slump hump protocol. The down arm's shoulder joint is resting and opening. The way in which your arms move in that smooth opposing way is what helps self-correct neck and shoulder pain and stiffness.

Okay! On to Day 8 when you're ready.

Day 8

Back in the saddle.

1. Alignment

2. Action: 10 TT

3. Appreciation

Did you take a rest day? Great! Now today you get to start up without drama or struggle. We stay with ten TT today as you practice coming back from a day off. Tomorrow, we'll add in the hamstring stretch.

Exercise promise interruption happens organically in life. In this thirty-day program, we orchestrate the rest day so you can practice starting and stopping without drama. When you have stoppage during life, you just do the same thing, AAA 10TT.

We will have another rest day soon. In the meantime, if you need a break, take one. If life happens and you get offtrack, just get back on when you're ready, ta-da. If you simply opted out for no reason, no worries, just AAA 10TT.

AAA goes a long way to taking the struggle out of exercise. AAA is the key to the starting and stopping with ease. A few things to consider about your AAA:

- Are you comfortable with when and where you are doing your practice?

- Do you have a regular time and space for it?

- Sometimes, after the first week, people realize that they could make this easier by doing it first thing in the morning when possible.

- I had a personal training client who was seventy-five years old and had been exercising regularly for fifty years. I asked her to what did she attribute her long-standing success. She said, "I always get it done first thing in the morning, before my brain wakes up and can talk me out of it."

- I have many clients who do their practice at the kitchen table with their morning coffee or tea. I have one client who does her Tush Tilts with her cat on her lap in the morning. I have another client who has a long commute so she does her thing at lunch break in her office. One more example is doing your stuff during your morning bathroom time. TT on the throne!

Tomorrow, we will be adding on a hamstring stretch to your routine. Until then, here's to standing strong and moving forward!

Jessica's Feedback

I am comfortable doing my exercises in the morning. Once they're done, they're done. Right now, I do them sitting on my bed. It's a great feeling of accomplishment when I complete my exercises at the time that I have chosen. Indeed, no drama.

Day 9

If you're already prepared to do your Hamstring Stretch, proceed with today's AAA. If you need to review the hamstring guidelines, you'll find them below. If you missed it, there is more hamstring info and pictures at the beginning of chapter 2.

1. Alignment

2. Action: 10TT, Hamstring Stretch

3. Appreciation

Today, we are adding a hamstring stretch to your routine. The hamstring muscle is the back of your thigh. Some general stretching guidelines:

- Be gentle. The stretch should feel small or medium. Never big. If you stretch too hard, your body will sometimes react by tightening up.

- Hold in a comfortable place for fifteen to thirty seconds.

- The hamstring stretch goes really well right after the Tush Tilts because the area gets a little warmed up and then muscle stretches easily.

Here are some positional options for stretching your hamstrings:

My favorite, the Famous Flop Over. Stand facing your bed, legs pretty straight, front of thighs touching the edge. Bend forward from the waist and let your upper body rest on the bed. You may feel this stretch from your back down to your heels. Remember gentle, hold for fifteen to thirty seconds.

Alternative Flop Over. You can do this almost anywhere. Stand facing your chair or toilet. Legs straight, bend from the waist, and put your hands on the seat. If you need more stretch, you can put your forearms on the seat. You can also do it by your desk, table, or counter. Legs pretty straight, then bend at the waist and support yourself on the surface in front of you. Play with this because stretching your hamstrings is fun to do almost anywhere.

Seated Hamstring Stretch. Sit in good posture. Straighten your right leg keeping your heel on the floor. That alone may get you the stretch. If not, stick your butt out a bit and see how that feels. You can also flex your foot, which may get you a calf stretch too, which is a good idea. Then try the other leg. Often your legs will feel this differently from side to side.

Sometimes, if your calves are pretty tight, that is where you will feel the stretch first and that's just fine. Your calf muscle is the back of the lower leg. Tight calf muscles contribute to knee, foot, and heel pain so it's great if you get some calf stretching done at this point. When your calves loosen up a bit, then your hamstrings will be more stretchable.

Try these, pick the one that works best for you and your body. Hold for fifteen to thirty seconds.

Voila!

Jessica's Feedback

I appreciate the variety of postures available for the flop over. I love these kinds of stretches especially because they are very effective for my sciatic flare-ups.

I noticed that you mentioned straight legs when bending. I bend or soften my knees, resisting the habit of locking them. Is that correct? *Cinder says yes, do what feels best to you.*

Yesterday, I had a phone meeting and after I popped, *yes* popped up and aligned with ease getting my exercises done. Aligning with journaling is challenging. I am easily distracted. It's funny, I am gaining appreciation for Nike's slogan "Just Do It." Who would've thunk it?

Day 10
Steady as She Goes

1. Alignment

2. Action: 10TT, Hamstring Stretch

3. Appreciation

As promised, we're gonna look more at ease and struggle.

Struggle is the opposite of ease. You can be doing nothing and be struggling. I'll bet you know what I mean by that. Struggle mostly comes from your mind. You might be having some of it as you approach this program. It's stuff in your head that makes this hard. Because really, what we're doing is not physically hard, but it's easy to make it feel that way.

Let's look at ease. You can work hard with ease. Do you know what I mean by that? For instance, I love boxing; I work hard with ease. I'm enjoying writing this book because I'm doing it with AAA. I'm only writing a page a day. AAA write a page. Ease. AAA is how you smooth out the path. Alignment is setting your mindset. Action must be small, small, small, and sweet. Then appreciate yourself as much as you can.

Tomorrow, we'll talk a bit about momentum and how it effects struggle and ease.

Jessica's Feedback

I caught myself projecting into the future. I felt fear of not making this experience a habit. Interestingly, I became aligned with action and being present by doing my exercises. Being prepared really helps. When I got up, I made sure to grab my tablet before I sat back down again, so journaling was not negotiable. Actually, it was, but I chose not to negotiate. *Good for me!*

Being aligned has been easier, remembering ease will help me get there, to not overthink and project into the future. There really is no ease there in those habits. As I write and read this page, I am able to breathe in ease! I totally get how doing nothing or the perception of doing nothing can be *the* struggle. Because the exercise is so simple, the structure really becomes what aligns me.

The acknowledgment of this being hard work has been very important; however, learning about ease and conscious alignment in relationship to exercise is a game changer for me.

Day 11

Appreciation and Momentum

1. Alignment

2. Action 10TT, Hamstring Stretch

3. Appreciation

Take a moment and appreciate yourself for still being here. Let's shine the spotlight on appreciation. Appreciating yourself will help you build momentum on this good-feeling fitness path. Let's face it. It's more normal to feel bad about your body than appreciative of the miracle that is you.

We are mostly influenced today into thinking there's something wrong—something wrong with ourselves and/or our bodies. Because I've been a personal trainer for decades, I've been hanging around in gym locker rooms for years. I noticed something interesting. Most women, no matter what they look like, are unhappy with their bodies. I have been off the diet and self-hatred roller coaster for almost thirty years. I often feel like one of the only women I know who actually likes herself.

If you practice appreciation of yourself, you will feel better and better, because whatever you put your attention on gets bigger. Appreciation puts you in alignment. Have you noticed that? Imagine using AAA over and over throughout your day. Using it into driving to work, using it into your next business meeting or phone call or whatever you're doing next.

The Stream of Well-Being

I heard "the stream of well-being" metaphor from Abraham-Hicks, and once again, I was thrilled to have words to put to what I know and teach. I believe there is a stream of well-being dominant in all aspects of my life. I have known that in relation to my body since I stopped dieting and hating myself all those decades ago. The stream is always there, but sometimes, I'm pinching myself off from it. Appreciation puts me in the stream and if I stay there long enough, I will gather the momentum of being aligned with well-being. Everything is easier from being aligned.

That is a side effect of the Easy Fitness system—that your experience of well-being increases. When you are in the stream of well-being and you'll know it because you'll feel good, appreciate yourself for being there. This will build good-feeling momentum for you. The better it gets, the better it gets. Momentum in a direction that feels good and is good for you!

Relax about this. It's normal to go in and out of the stream. The most important thing right now is that the time we spend together feels lovely and friendly. We are in the stream for a few minutes right now, and it is good.

Tomorrow, we will add a small easy good-feeling next step.

Jessica's Feedback

Today was an easy exercise "action" day and a challenging alignment day. It took a few tries to settle into my tilts because I was distracted by thoughts about my choices yesterday. Choices that didn't have anything to do with my exercises but were not in alignment and definitely not in appreciation. It's that icky feeling that I could have done more or different. *Ahhh* . . . everything in front, nothing behind. I appreciate that I took this moment to get to right now. I felt the shift to alignment when I became present, shifting my focus to what is in front of me.

What is in front is that I prepared myself for exercise without hesitation this morning. Filling my water container and grabbing my journal without a second thought. I am noticing that yesterday's choices are mellowing, washing away. I acknowledge that I am motivated and am doing my best. I appreciate that I am focused and motivated to pay attention to what is in front of me. Opening my own stream, creating alignment, creating appreciation. It is indeed good!

Day 12
A Few Shoulder Rolls

To do a Shoulder Roll intentionally, move your shoulder back, up, forward, and around. Repeat and reverse.

1. Alignment

2. Action: 10TT, Hamstring, Shoulder Rolls 2 back, 2 front

3. Appreciation

Tomorrow, we will add the Swimmer. Shoulder rolls get you ready for that.

You are on the leading edge with this program. The leading edge is doing something different. Something most folks are not doing. Easy Fitness is the leading edge because you are learning how to use exercise as a way to take really good care of yourself. Most other fitness avenues are an obvious or subtle way to beat yourself up. AAA puts you on the leading edge. Most people take action without knowing it's better to be in alignment first.

Remember, our second key is, "Don't give a damn about what anyone else thinks."

This Easy Fitness path requires that you feel good first (alignment) and then take your small step (action). Most other programs are going for the feel good after you get your "results." (Results that never come actually, so you never feel good.)

There are more benefits from feeling good first other than just feeling good. When you get used to taking action from a place of feeling good first, you will never be stuck waiting to feel motivated. As a matter of fact, when you learn to take action from a place of feeling good emotionally and mentally (alignment), you're next steps will feel inspired and easy. You will not need motivation anymore.

Motivation is what we do when we are taking an action from a place of worry about what might happen.

Inspiration is what we do when we take an action after being aligned with a good-feeling thought.

The moment you think that good-feeling thought (that is how we've asked you to get into alignment), you are in the stream of well-being. The ideas that come to you when you are in alignment (or in the stream) are inspired. The action you take while you are in the stream of well-being is inspired and leveraged. No need for motivation when you are taking inspired action. This is a leading edge way of thinking about your health and happiness. This is the foundation of Easy Fitness.

These words help explain the path, but nothing teaches like living the experience. Relax and enjoy these minutes that we are together each day. Let your inspired Easy Fitness path unfold in a perfect way for you.

See you tomorrow for a swimmer lesson.

Jessica's Feedback

(This is so rich and wonderful today)

Cinder, I have been using alignment as a mental exercise. Yes, the good-feeling thought came naturally until today. Read further . . . your input would be helpful.

Wonky Saturday. Actually, I started feeling wonky last night. When I woke up this morning, my mental alignment eluded me. I was distracted and felt on edge. After taking a two-hour nap, I felt resistance big time because it was almost noon. All of those old messages started flooding in. Quitting is not an option; not keeping my promise is not an option. I felt very emotional as I sat on the side of my bed. Coaxing myself, just do Shoulder Rolls. I let the tears of resistance up and out releasing those old stories. Before I knew it, I was doing my tilts and ending with the hamstring flop. I did it. I did it late, I did it out of sequence. I did it in a funk, and *I did it*! If this isn't being on the leading edge of well-being, I don't know what is.

I did not feel good first and was able to find alignment as I knew I would feel better by trying. Just trying. Just try helped me to stay put long enough to align with the idea of doing my AAA. The feel good came with the accomplishment of doing what I said I would do.

Day 13
Swimmers!

1. Alignment

2. Action: 10TT, Hamstring, Shoulder Rolls/Swimmers

3. Appreciation

Today, I'd like you to consider adding in a few Swimmers (start with 3 or 5). If you missed the full instructions and benefits at the beginning of this chapter, you can go back and read or try these abbreviated instructions. If something hurts or is unclear, go back to the full instruction.

The Swimmer

- Sit on the edge of your chair so your hands can hang down.

- Good sitting posture is ninety-degree leg position with your ankles under your knees, rib cage lifted, and your head being a natural extension of your spine.

- Now raise your right hand in the air as if you wanted to be called on by the teacher. Modification: You can have your palm facing front. Or you can have your palm facing in. One position may feel friendlier than the other. Try and see.

- We want your arms to move as if they were straight arm levers moving up and down in front of your body. The swimming motion comes as one is going up, one is coming down. Your straight arms should pass each other at about chest height and reach their up/down destinations at the same time.

- Pause with one hand up in the air and one hand down at your side, then switch the positions.

- Move deliberately and smoothly.

- Here's how the muscles are working. At the top of the motion, the back of your shoulder is getting stronger at the same time as the front of that shoulder is mobilized or stretching. The down arm's shoulder joint is resting and opening. The way in which your arms move in a smooth opposing way is what helps self-correct neck and shoulder pain and stiffness.

- I suggest you try three or five of these today.

Happy swimming!

Day 14

You have been exercising consistently for fourteen days! Yay you!

I'm treating Days 7, 14, 21, and 28 as a reason for talking about rest days. We are going to talk about how to find your way when you take a rest day.

I give recommendations that I believe will be pretty good for most folks, but at this point, you will need to be paying attention to your body and making some decisions. Remember, in the beginning, I told you that *you* would become your own exercise expert! We're starting that now.

Today, you might decide to take a rest day. If you haven't taken one yet, I suggest you do and see how you feel about it. Part of taking a rest day is starting back up the next day.

The starting back up is an empowering moment. How many times have you gotten stuck about exercise? Not knowing where to start. Or getting offtrack with it, not being able to get back to it. Most people have no ease about exercise. Most people are afraid if they stop, they'll never start again. Lots of people never even start.

That's what's so great about Easy Fitness. This Easy Fitness path circumvents all that traditional fitness crap that keeps people stuck and frustrated. With Easy Fitness, we make this exercise thing simple and doable, so you don't have to worry about stopping and not being able to start again.

So take a rest day. Enjoy it. Know that a rest day is just as important as an exercise day. It's good for your body. It's great to practice stopping and starting because starting and stopping is a natural phenomenon in life when it comes to exercise. Relax. Rest.

Next week, you will learn all about how to add on to your practice in the perfect right way for you!

3

Miracle Knee and Our Third Week

Finding Your Way

This week, you will be learning to listen to your body. Being able to hear your body's wisdom will make you your own best expert. Remember, our success formula is *you* doing what *you* say you will do about exercise. You decide. We will give you ways and means to increase your AAA if it feels right. Also this week, we will learn a brilliant knee healing small step, an energy experiment and a third key. All these aspects will fold right into what you are already doing.

How to know *if* it's time to add on. Most of you are probably at AAA 10TT, Hamstring stretch, and three to five Swimmers. Here are some things to consider as you think about adding on to your routine.

How do you feel physically while you're doing your AAA?

- Does it feel friendly to your body?

- Does your body feel like a willing participant?

- Does something feel not quite right?

How do you feel physically after?

- Energized?

- Tired?

- Fine?

The answers to those questions determine where you're at and what to do next. For instance, if the above routine is feeling fine and friendly, you're on the right track; you can add on if you want. If not, you have to back something off. Maybe take out the Swimmers and do Shoulder Rolls. Maybe you want to do the Shoulder Rolls and then the Swimmers 'cause it feels better that way. Maybe three Swimmers is okay, but five is too many.

Stay present and notice how your body feels during and right after AAA. Make a decision about moving forward. Give it a try. See how you feel. If you are feeling eager and energized, you might want to add a couple repetitions of TT or Swimmers.

- *Always add in small increments.*

- *Remember we're building a foundation that you will use forever so take it slow*

- *Pay attention*

- *Course correct when needed*

Relaxed Expansion. The nuts and bolts of increasing your AAA exercise safely and sanely. Are you ready to increase? Yes, if what you're doing feels easy and doable on a regular basis. If you feel relaxed and maybe even happy when you think about your current exercise promise, then it's time to think about how to add on. There is *no rush*. Wait for it to feel right before you expand your AAA.

Relaxed Expansion Terms:

Repetitions or Reps. The number of times you do the actual movement

Sets. A group of reps with a rest in between

Frequency. How often

Intensity. The actual amount of effort or circumstances that effect effort

Duration. The length of time

Here are some alternatives for moving forward:

- Reps: Increase reps, add one or two of everything or some things.

- Sets: Add a second set. When adding a second set, you do less reps and work up to two sets of ten

- Frequency: Do your second set(s) at another time

- Intensity: You can squeeze harder or add reps or decrease rest between sets

- Duration: Add your second set at the same time and you increase length of time exercising

There are a million different combos of the above. After you think it through, you try it and see how it feels. If it feels doable but not quite as easy, you're on the right track.

You might try different combos to see what's best for you. For instance, if your mornings are crowded, you might want to do a second set of everything later in the day. Sometimes, it's wonderful to do a flop over hamstring before you go to bed.

Figuring this out and knowing how flexible you can be about it will give you freedom—freedom to choose what's exactly right for you! You can always come back to this page and find a way to make the exercise fit into your life.

In the coming week, we're going to be paying attention to your body's response to all this. We'll be learning the difference between your body's voice of wisdom and your monkey mind. Everybody's got both, and they're easy to tell apart.

Also, this week we will be suggesting the Miracle Knee exercise on Day 17! Here are full instructions. Abbreviated instruction will be included on Day 17.

The Miracle Knee

The number one recommended rehab exercise for knees is a quad set. Your quadriceps muscle (or quad) is the group of muscles in the front of your thigh, above your knee.

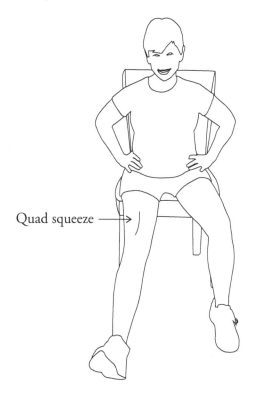

Quad squeeze

The Miracle Knee

Having these muscles stronger is the key to supporting your knee.

I have been helping folks get fit for more than twenty years. What my clients noticed was when they did this simple sitting exercise, their knees felt better right away. It was like a miracle. And so they named this exercise the Miracle Knee Exercise. If you do it, you can expect a knee miracle!

Let's try it together right now…

Start sitting in the ninety-degree position. Straighten the right leg keeping your heel on the ground, foot relaxed. Put your right hand on your thigh above your knee if you can reach.

Now straighten your leg a little bit more by pushing the back of your knee toward the floor. Some knees will lock or go past locked (mine does), according to doctors, this is okay. You decide what feels ok for you.

What you should feel under your hand is the quad muscle shortening or bunching up. That's the muscle contracting. Hold for two seconds, then release. Voila! You have just done the Miracle Knee! Be sure to NOT squeeze your butt.

Always breathe during the contraction. Counting the seconds out loud can help you remember to breathe. Sometimes, you can feel your kneecap moving up toward your waist. That's fine. If this hurts your knee, don't push down so hard. Once you feel how to get the contraction you can modify the intensity of the squeeze. Squeeze intensity scale: easy, medium, hard. Go easy.

Now try the left leg, notice any differences. Find the contraction, then modify the intensity.

I suggest you start with two or three repetitions on each leg. How you add on to this exercise is by increasing the holding time. So you might start with two 2-sec holds on each leg. Then move to two 5-sec holds on each leg. We cap it at ten second holds. *Breathing* during the holds is really important. Remember, counting out loud will make breathing easy.

We are adding this knee healing super power small step on Day 17 along with more great knee healing information on Day 21.

Day 15

1. Alignment

2. Action: 10TT, Hamstring, Shoulder/3–5 Swimmers

3. Appreciation

The Energy Experiment

Today, before you do your practice, check in about your energy. Does your energy feel low, medium, or high? Don't think too hard about it. Just notice. Then do your practice. Then check in again after AAA and see if your energy changed. Often, you will find that AAA will give you an energy boost. Check it out for yourself. The energy experiment can be different from one day to the next. It can even change as the day proceeds.

The takeaway here is to note that sometimes, a little Easy Fitness break can improve your energy in the moment. Good to know! I have clients who use a little Easy Fitness AAA all through their day to keep their energy even and good.

You can add the energy check in before and after AAA. It's a good way to make a habit of listening to your body. And it only takes a moment. Tomorrow, you will learn all about hearing your body's voice of wisdom.

Day 16

Voice of Wisdom

1. Alignment

2. Action: 10TT, Hamstring Stretch, 3–5 Swimmers

3. Appreciation

After today, I will no longer be putting in numbers because you will be determining what's right for you! Today's lesson is so exciting because when you learn to distinguish your voice of wisdom from the other voice in your head, you will be able to find your next step with more ease. You will be getting good at determining what's right for you. The other voice that we have in our heads (not voice of wisdom) can sometimes be referred to as monkey mind. Monkey mind is a Buddhist term describing that aspect of our minds that is chattering at us constantly as it swings from doubt to worry to fear and back again. It's a normal human thing to have both voice of wisdom and monkey mind. Here's how you tell them apart.

Monkey mind thoughts are loud in your brain, insistent and repetitive. If you've got a thought you're thinking over and over, it's probably monkey mind.

Voice of wisdom is quiet, gentle, patient, and often has a lovely easy humor.

You can tell what thoughts you're listening to by how you feel.

When you are listening to monkey mind, you might feel anxious, worried, bad about yourself, or any version of those.

When you are listening to voice of wisdom, you will feel relaxed, hopeful/optimistic, present and/or "All is well."

When you do AAA, you are training to essentially feel relaxed and good about what you are doing. It's a way to get used to listening to voice of wisdom. Isn't it nice to know you have been connected to your voice of wisdom?

Today, if you're game, notice when you are feeling a bit out of sorts—worried, doubtful, anxious, down on yourself—pause, smile, and relax knowing it's just monkey mind. If you can find the smile and relax, then try a quick TT and appreciate yourself for the shift you just made.

There's nothing wrong with monkey mind; it's a normal human thing. Actually, learning to recognize monkey mind is pretty cool because it leads you to AAA and voice of wisdom.

It's really normal to have monkey mind when you are doing something new.

Listening to voice of wisdom puts you in the stream of well-being where all is well. A great and wonderful benefit of being in the stream of well-being is that from there, you will often be inspired with good-feeling ideas. The actions that are inspired from the stream of well-being ideas will often feel leveraged and easy.

Listening to monkey mind pinches you off from the stream. You can tell by how you feel—ornery, anxious, angry, or despairing to name a few. But it's no big deal. Once you notice you are not in the stream, relax, smile, and shift. This really only works if you catch it early. If monkey mind's got a pretty good hold, hang on it'll be over soon.

Learning to shift from monkey mind to voice of wisdom will not only make exercise easier, but you will notice life getting easier too. The more ease you are experiencing, the more energy you will have for your life in general.

Jessica's Feedback

Voice of wisdom, man did I need to read this page today. I woke up feeling unsure, my confidence felt low, I could feel the beginning of a shut down and then I remembered that I needed to AAA. I actually said out loud, "I am not quitting!" I pushed myself literally out of bed and did my AAA.

Day 17
Miracle Knee Day!

1. Alignment

2. Action TT, Hamstring, Shoulder/Swimmer, Miracle Knee

3. Appreciation

I have included Miracle Knee instruction here. Try 2 repetitions of 2 second holds on each leg today, only if it feels right to you.

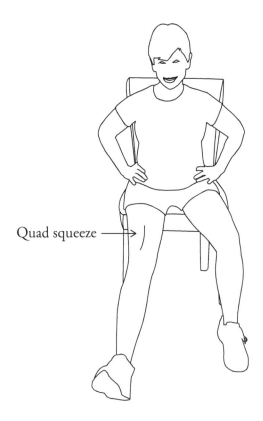

Quad squeeze →

The Miracle Knee

The number one recommended rehab exercise for knees is a quad set. Your Quadriceps muscle (or quad) is the group of muscles in the front of your thigh, above your knee. Having these muscles stronger is the key to supporting your knee.

My clients noticed that when they did this simple sitting exercise, their knees felt better right away. It was like a miracle. And so they named this exercise the Miracle Knee Exercise. If you do it, you can expect a knee miracle!

Start sitting in the ninety-degree position. Straighten the right leg keeping your heel on the ground, foot relaxed. Put your right hand on your thigh above your knee if you can reach.

Now straighten your leg a little bit more by pushing the back of your knee toward the floor. Some knees will lock or go past locked (mine does), according to doctors, this is okay. You decide what feels okay for you.

What you should feel under your hand is the quad muscle shortening or bunching up. That's the muscle contracting. Hold for two seconds, then release. Voila! You have just done the Miracle Knee!

Always breathe during the contraction. Counting the seconds out loud can help you remember to breathe. Sometimes, you can feel your kneecap moving up toward your waist. That's fine. If this hurts your knee, don't push down so hard. Once you feel how to get the contraction, you can modify the intensity of the squeeze. Squeeze intensity scale: easy, medium, hard. Go easy.

Now try the left leg, notice any differences. Find the contraction, then modify the intensity. I suggest you start with two or three repetitions on each leg. How you add on to this exercise is by increasing the holding time. So you might start with two 2-sec holds on each leg. The move to two 5-sec holds on each leg. We cap it at ten second holds. *Breathing* during the holds is really important. Remember, counting out loud will make breathing easy.

Day 18
Checking In

1. Alignment

2. Action: TT, Hamstring Stretch, Shoulder Rolls/Swimmers, Miracle Knee

3. Appreciation

This is a check-in day. I appreciate you for hanging in there with this! Together, we have designed a small and powerful exercise routine for you, which you have been doing consistently for more than two weeks! Brilliant! How's it feeling? Easy? Medium? Hard?

Can you differentiate struggle from ease? Remember, struggle usually comes from your mind. If you are feeling less than good, i.e., struggling, you might be listening to monkey mind thoughts. Notice, relax, smile if you can, then AAA. If you are experiencing pretty much ease about this, what do you notice about that? Do you look forward to how it feels to be in AAA? Do you like the feeling of accomplishment?

Are you using AAA anywhere else in your life?

What are you noticing physically?

Some folks feel more connected to their bodies and more specifically their butts, as they proceed with this course.

Some people find it's easier to get in and out of the car or to get up from a chair or to do chores.

What are you noticing?

Is there anything that needs adjusting in your routine?

Appreciate yourself for the care you are taking of yourself.

Appreciate yourself for learning a new skill.

Appreciate yourself for _____ (fill in the blank)

See you tomorrow!

Jessica's Feedback

I will speak to what caused today's struggle. (I am in deep gratitude and appreciation for figuring this out in the middle of monkey mind). One of your questions was about using AAA principles anywhere else in my life. I use alignment a lot in my life both mentally and physically. Yesterday, I started off feeling accomplished and then when I got to a family gathering, I stepped back into the habit of sitting and asking others to help or serve me. How can I talk about my progress and excitement and demonstrate inactivity at the same time? I know in earlier writing you have reminded me to not worry about what others think. Yesterday, I didn't realize that that was playing in my subconscious. That is until this morning when it popped up loud and clear. Wondering and worrying about how others saw me, how can I be so happy in an inactive, no, low active body. I was so unconscious that I stepped into an unconscious action. I wanted to get a head start walking; my cousin was walking with me, and I wasn't present. I just wanted to get to my car; I just wanted to sit down. Here's what I missed out on because of this habit. I missed hugs good-bye from my friends and family. I had not realized how that habit has affected my connections. I am in so much appreciation for not letting the monkey mind continue to affect me today. I have the opportunity to learn and do something different next time.

The exercise feels easy and effective. I find myself using the tilts and yes, definitely, my butt every time I go from a sitting to a standing position. Where I have noticed a lot of change is in using my butt specifically to gain momentum to stand. As I feel my butt push me higher off the seat, I focus on ease to get me to standing and then patience to get steady. Appreciating myself for not giving up.

Day 19

A Third Key

1. Alignment

2. Action: TT, Hamstring Stretch, Shoulder Rolls/Swimmers, Miracle Knee

3. Appreciation

Today, I'm introducing you to a third key, and it's really good news. Let me remind you of the first two keys:

1. Nothing behind, everything in front.

2. Don't give a damn about what anyone else thinks.

And here is the third key:

3. You never get it done, so you can't get it wrong!

I learned this key from Abraham-Hicks, and once again, these words fit me perfectly. Here's what I mean with this key. Life is always changing. You (and me too) are always on your way somewhere. We are always learning and growing. We never get it done; we never stop moving forward. We are never static. That's the good news. It means you are alive!

Because things are always changing and/or expanding (you're never done till you croak), there's nothing wrong with where you are. You always have another shot at it, so you can't get it wrong! Aren't you happy to know that? When I find myself worrying about a wrong turn that I took or a misstep with work or relationships, I remember that it's never done and I'll have another chance. Phew. I can't get it wrong. No matter what happens with AAA or your exercise, relax; there's always another shot at it if you want.

When I really started to understand and embrace this key, I was able to relax into my life. I noticed that even when I had something wonderful happening, I was expectant about more wonderful stuff (you never get it done). Expansion comes as you grow things you like and as you figure out what to do instead of something you didn't like. I find myself embracing the expansion that is a natural part of life.

The true benefit in this key is that you can relax into your life, right where you are, knowing that since you never get it done, you can give it another shot later or tomorrow. You can't get it wrong 'cause you never get it done. There's always more growth and expansion. There's always another try. We are always learning and growing. All is well. (Note: Monkey mind will not want you to learn or believe this. Voice of wisdom knows it absolutely.)

Can you see how this key could change your experience of fitness forever? There are so many clichés that would fit here: Life is a journey, enjoy the journey, smell the roses, change is good, change is inevitable, and there are no mistakes . . . The best feeling by-product of this third key is the feeling of all is well.

That's what this book is really all about. Living each day with as much ease and joy as possible. Just take one day at a time. Do a little exercise, AAA as much as possible during the day. Appreciate yourself, know that all is well.

Relax, squeeze your butt, and smell the roses.

Day 20
Smooth Sailing...

1. Alignment

2. Action: TT, Hamstring Stretch, Shoulder Rolls/Swimmers, Miracle Knee

3. Appreciation

We're gonna stay with these exercises for a few days. We'll be learning one more exercise category soon.

Right now you could be doing:

- Everything most days

- Some most days

- All at once in the morning, noon or night

- Breaking it up during the day

- Less or more depending on how you feel

- Adding to your practice or not

The skill here is starting to hear what your body wants and needs. If you don't know, try a little something and then see how you feel.

Jessica's Feedback

Exercising and practicing flexibility has been a consistent and interesting experiment. Since Wednesday, I have done butt tilts, flop overs, shoulder rolls, and swimmers in all kinds of orders and at various times together and broken up. I am enjoying the flexibility, moving without punishment, and tons of appreciation. I even shared the AAAs with a friend of mine who is adding a yoga practice to her life. She loved how inspiring it is. I say it often, think it more than that and find that I'm using my thighs and glutes differently when preparing to stand up. I am noticing that my patience is increasing as I stabilize myself, even though I'm sore more often, the feeling of accomplishment is big.

I am realizing that putting conditions on my exercise program only prevents me from being creative about my exercises. Allowing myself to be creative leads me to appreciation. Using AAA at any given moment helps me to stay in check in mode. Today, all is well.

Exercise doesn't feel like coasting yet, though I'm able to begin exercise with ease. I enjoyed reading about Day 20's flexibility and appreciation for every effort and accomplishment. The reality is that alignment in whatever I am feeling will get me to the next step. These tools have helped me in many daily accomplishments, which has heightened my appreciation.

Back to Cinder

More on smooth sailing.

Remember that sometimes your thoughts will get in the way of your practice. You can mostly tell when that is happening because you might feel stressed, worried, frustrated, sad, or angry to name a few. When struggle happens, relax and know it's normal. Smile at yourself if you can. Squeeze your butt if you can, just for fun. Get on with your day.

If you can't break the struggle spell, don't worry. Wait for a moment later on when you're feeling good, then squeeze your butt. Struggle is a normal human experience. Here's a saying I learned long ago that I love and find very useful. I also like it because it's funny. Warning: curse word included.

"Just 'cause you step in a bucket of shit, doesn't mean you should jump up and down in it."

So if you're having a moment of struggle, or if it's gotten bigger than a moment, distract yourself if you can. These things might mitigate struggle:

- Pet your dog or cat

- Listen to a happy song if you can find one that doesn't piss you off

- Look at something pleasing to you (nature is great for this)

- Think of someone who is easy for you to appreciate

- Watch *Big Bang Theory*

- You can take a nap, meditate, or go to bed

On taking a nap or going to bed, as I fall asleep, I bring to mind something simple to appreciate, my pillow, my home, my dog. I fall asleep in appreciation. When you awake, your vibration (which will influence your thoughts) will be where you left it. Hence the argument for falling asleep in appreciation.

When you awake, find something simple to appreciate. See how long you can stay there before the worries and chores of the day take over. Sometimes, I don't even make it through my first cup of coffee. Some days, I'm there most of the day. But I don't worry because I know I can't get it wrong 'cause I never get it done!

AAA is meant to pre-pave your fitness path into a path of less struggle. That is why it's so important to creating a good-feeling fitness practice. That's also why we encourage "first thing in the morning" in case struggle jumps on early in the day.

Your experience with your exercise practice will most likely be a little different from day to day. That's okay. It gives you a chance to practice navigating. Remember: You never get it done so you can't get it wrong!

Tomorrow is a rest day if you want one. And I'm going to give you some magic knee healing tips!

Day 21
Heal Your Knee 1-2-3!

Wow, three weeks! You rock!

Today can be a rest day if you want a break. Remember, stopping and starting is normal and a good skill to practice.

Did you know I'm an expert in helping plus-size people with knee pain? In my decades of working with folks with big bodies, I noticed that most had "knee issues." Over time, I discovered what worked the easiest and best to help with the knee pain. All the exercises we've done so far are part of the Heal Your Knee 1-2-3 program. If you have knee pain, look for improvement. You might already be noticing less pain or greater mobility.

Today, I'm gonna share with you three mistakes most people make that hurt their knees and what to do instead. I know at least one person whose knee pain cleared completely when she followed these tips.

Three Mistakes that Can Hurt Your Knees Even When You're Not Moving

Knee pain can often get in the way moving forward with life let alone an exercise program. If you have knee pain, you're in the right place because healing knees is something we help people with every day.

If you have knee pain, you're not alone. In the United States, 19.4 million doctor visits each year are about knee pain. Now imagine the people that don't go to the doctor, that's a lot of knee pain.

Today, we're gonna give you three easy ways to reduce knee pain by pointing out three mistakes most people make and what to do about them.

Many movements put pressure on your knees; over time, this can lead to discomfort and serious pain. Even something as simple as how you sit, stand, and sleep unknowingly contribute to knee pain.

Mistake number one. Sitting with your knees tucked way underneath you for long periods of time. You put unnecessary strain on your knees when you sit like this.

The Fix. Ninety-degree rule: Sit with your knees over your ankles so you have a ninety-degree bend. If/when you find yourself sitting with your feet tucked under you at your desk, undo it. Just keep noticing and changing. Bonus: The extra moving back and forth is good for the joint . . . motion is lotion.

I have a client who was always stiff and sore when she stood up at work. When she used the ninety-degree rule, that stiff unsteady feeling went away. Now she is getting up from her desk with ease and even using the stairs instead of the elevator. As her pain decreases and her mobility increases, she gets more enthusiastic and productive at work.

Mistake number two. Standing with your knees locked. Your knee is a hinge joint; think of it like a car door hinge. If the car door is open as far as it goes, doesn't it feel like you might break it if you keep pushing? Well, that's what it's like when you are standing with your knees locked—the hinge is at the end range and then you push it. The locked position also makes your knee joint responsible for holding your body weight instead of your muscles.

The Fix: When you are standing, soften your knees. Try it now, stand and let your weight sit mostly on your heels and balls of feet, knees soft (unlocked). It's that easy. Go from locked to unlocked a few time and notice what it feels like. Bonus: Gently squeeze your butt muscles as you unlock your knees so those muscles can hold your body weight.

Mistake number three. Sleeping in the fetal position (I know, keep reading).

The Fix: Reduce knee pain while you sleep. Really? Really! So if you are a side sleeper, keep your knees at ninety degrees or even straight (sleep in an "L") instead of fetal. Could it be that simple? No one tells you this but the more time you spend with your legs straight, the less strain on your knees. If you sleep on your back, then your legs are straight and you are golden.

The only thing you need to implement these tips is awareness, so when you notice you are doing one of the mistakes, simply undo it.

4

Your Get Up and Go

We have been happily plugging along, one day at a time, building positive momentum on your Easy Fitness path. I hope you are noticing more ease in the rest of your life too. AAA is a powerful tool. Over the next week, you will see how the Easy Fitness success formula (Doing what I said I would do about exercise, consistently and without struggle) is working. Actually, how *you* are working it! Take a moment right now to appreciate yourself and your path.

On Day 23, I will be introducing you to the Easy Fitness Make a Choice Formula. This formula was born out of my work with my mentor and coach Dr. Maria Nemeth. She uses similar words in her ground-breaking book and program *Mastering Life's Energies* to guide her clients and readers to act with clarity, focus, ease, and grace.

A big moment this week comes on Day 24 as you learn how to make getting up from any chair easier. Getting up from a chair may seem like a big chore right now, but you'll have ways to make it instantly easier. Eventually, you may even find yourself getting up for fun and exercise! You're gonna love how your heel-butt connection helps with getting up.

Right now, I'm introducing you to two Easy Fitness small steps called the Heel Tap and the Football Huddler. These small powerful steps not only build strength and flexibility, but they also make get ups easier and solve two big mobility problems. Don't you love how much bang for your buck you get from these small step exercises? I will tell you how to do them and what they do for you next. We will revisit these two exercises as we approach the get up later in the week.

Heel Taps decrease knee pain and increase mobility instantly.

The Heel Tap is one of the exercises in my Heal Your Knee 1-2-3 program. Heel Taps strengthen the front (quad muscle) and the back (hamstring muscle) of your thigh. At the same time, the bending and straightening moves your knee in a friendly way that helps lubricate the joint because motion is lotion! A tiny tilt in the Heel Tap keeps your back safe throughout the exercise while it builds your core strength. The Heel Tap builds leg strength and increases mobility in the knee joint.

The Heel Tap can be added into AAA, but it's even more useful than that because you can use it to solve this mobility problem: *You know how after you've been sitting for a while and then you get up, your knees might feel stiff, sore, and hardly able to hold you? Doing a few Heel Taps before you stand often resolves that problem because motion is lotion.* Here's how you do the Heel Tap, give it a try:

Heel Tap with a Tiny Tilt:

1. Sit in ninety-degree rule with upright posture

2. Do a small pelvic tilt (tiny tilt) and hold it gently

3. Straighten your right leg tapping your heel

4. Return to start position, relaxing the pelvic tilt

5. Repeat on the other leg

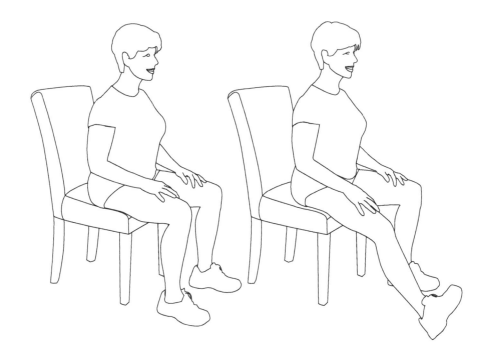

The Heel Tap

The Football Huddler position decreases back pain and increases mobility instantly.

You know how sometimes when you're walking the outside of your hips can start to ache or get tight? Next thing you know, you need to sit for a bit. Sometimes, it makes you afraid to go places where you might not be able to find a seat. The Football Huddler back stretch solves this problem with no sitting required.

You might think this walking hip pain is coming from your hips, but it's often caused by your low back tightening up. The best fix is to sit for a few seconds. If you catch it when it first starts, even ten seconds of sitting will help. Big mistake many people make is to just keep walking when this is happening. The pain only gets worse if you keep going. You must find an interrupt. Sitting is a great way to interrupt the pain cycle.

But what if there's nowhere to sit? Football Huddler to the rescue! Getting into the Football Huddler position relieves the strain on your low back, allowing you to continue walking with less or no hip pain. Use the Football Huddler early and often when there's no place to sit so you can get where you're going with less pain and drama. Here's how you do it:

- Stand with your feet spread pretty wide.

- Bend your knees a bit as you put your hands on your thighs

- Lean forward slightly as you stick your butt out a little

- Keep your eyes forward

- Imagine how the players look in a football huddle

This is the Football Huddler position. If you feel like it, next time you're up and about, give this stretching position a try. You can even do a tiny TT when you are in the position. Give that a try too.

Football Huddler gives your back a rest, relieves that outer hip pain, and sometimes you can feel a stretch in your back as well. You can hold the position for a few seconds then squeeze your butt as you come back to upright. Then continue your walk. When you have pain, use this early and often. Eventually, you will walk further and further with less pain!

The Football Huddler position and the Heel Tap will come into play this week as we learn about getting up from any seat with some ease. Until then, use these two movements to bring more ease and comfort into your everyday activities.

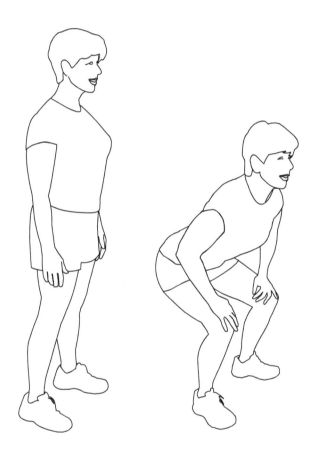

Football Huddler

Moving on to Day 22!

Day 22

1. Alignment

2. Action: TT, Hamstrings, Shoulder Rolls/Swimmers, Miracle Knee

3. Appreciation

Doing what I said I would do about exercise consistently and without struggle.

Let's look at the above sentence again. It is the Easy Fitness success formula that we introduced in the Setup. We're going to see how your Easy Fitness keys blend perfectly with this formula. You will notice how well you're doing!

In this book, I helped you get started, but at this point you are probably finding your own way. Deciding what to do, how much, when, where. You are deciding when to rest. When to take it easy, when to push. You are deciding what *you say you will do* about exercise. Because you are deciding, it makes the follow through seem like the next logical step. Boom. Nothing behind, everything in front.

Consistently! We've got that going on too. It's easier to be consistent with a practice that you are choosing the parameters of. Keep in mind that this Easy Fitness path is one of small steps and friendly feeling physical movements. It doesn't matter what anyone else is saying or what "the experts" say. You are the expert on your body. This freedom fuels your consistency. Don't give a damn about what anyone else thinks.

Without struggle? Well, you might be struggling some. It's a pretty normal human thing to struggle. What we're really learning here is to keep it to a minimum. Catch it early. If you can catch the feeling of struggle early, then you can often switch to AAA and squeeze your butt. Within your AAA practice itself, struggle is minimized.

Take a moment and look to see if you have been experiencing struggle. How do you know? What do you experience when you struggle? Is it anxiety? Frustration? Sadness? Anger? Distraction? Apathy? You want to catch struggle in the early subtle stages whenever possible. Identifying your personal experience will help you interrupt it. Think of the rumble strips on the highway. When you hit them, you know you need to get back in your lane, or go off the road. Knowing your personal experience of struggle is like your rumble strip.

You can't fix a *big* struggle from where you notice it (that's why we recommend catching it early). When you realize that struggle is having its way with you, relax. Say "later gator" to whatever you were thinking about and move on to something else. Think of something else for a while. This will take some focus. You can always take a nap. Then try again later or tomorrow. Don't worry, you never get it done so you can't get it wrong. Let this key soothe the struggle. There's always later or tomorrow. For today, practice doing what you said you would do about exercise consistently and without struggle.

Jessica's Feedback

I am learning how to treat exercise as a game, challenging myself in mind and body. A place where I can ask questions and change rules to meet me where I'm at.

Time . . . *hmmmmm*. Sitting with this thought, I am reminded about the importance of preparation. Having what I need at hand helps me to move out of struggle. I also remembered how "time" trips me up. Allowing flexibility takes the time expectation out of the equation. I also appreciate that redirecting the small struggle is much different than redirecting the big struggle. I was reminded of how I've trained my dog. When I catch his behavior early, it is much easier to manage than when his behavior is bigger.

When a big struggle has presented itself to me in the past, I gave up. Now I am learning to intuitively try again. Sometimes later in the day, sometimes the next day.

Day 23

1. Alignment

2. Action: TT, Hamstrings, Shoulder Rolls/Swimmers, Miracle Knee

3. Appreciation

Yesterday, you saw how well you were doing with the Easy Fitness success formula: Doing what I said I would do about exercise, consistently and without struggle. Today, you're going to learn the Easy Fitness Make a Choice Formula. It's a tool you can use when you are having trouble deciding what to do today about exercise. Don't you love the freedom in this program? *You* get to decide what *you* say you will do.

Here are some common scenarios that you may run into:

- You might not feel well, what do you do about your exercise?

- You might want to skip a day . . . is that all right?

- You might be so pressed for time that you don't feel like you have a minute.

- You have an injury.

- Fill in your own scenario.

What comes up for you some days when you think about your exercise practice? Sometimes you're sure what to do, sometimes you're not sure. Here's a tool to use when you are not clear about your next step. Ask yourself this question:

What would a person who is willing to be happy and healthy do today?

Answer that question. To exercise or not to exercise? Do more or do less? Look for the answer that makes you relax. Reach for the feeling of relief or certainty or clarity. Sometimes, the answer will be rest or move or take a nap or just squeeze your butt and move on. (PS you can replace happy and healthy if they don't land for you. I have some clients who prefer to say "who is willing to practice exquisite self-care," "who is willing to be in the stream of well-being.") Note the use of the word *willing*. Remember, we learned earlier that you can be willing to do what you don't want to do, what you don't know how to do or what you're afraid to do. You are always willing about something.

When you answer this question, you have made a choice. Now line up with your choice.

If you have chosen to exercise, proceed with ease. If you have chosen to rest, revel in it. The worst thing is to make a choice and then second-guess yourself. You'll know when you're doing that because you will feel bad in some way—anxious, mad at yourself, sad, angry, or, or, or.

Remember, this is a journey, a process. You are evolving into this exercise thing. You can never get it wrong because you can always try again later or tomorrow. There is no absolute destination (like weight loss) in Easy Fitness, only journey. You will always be evolving with this. Do you feel the freedom? You can't get it wrong 'cause you never get it done.

I suggest that you write the Easy Fitness Make a Choice Formula on a Post-it or index card or widget and ponder it. Copy it precisely as it's written then adjust the adjectives if you want to. You don't need to only use the question when you are uncertain. Practice using it for fun. Notice happy comes first.

What would a person who is willing to be happy and healthy do today?

- Answer the question

- Do the answer

- Enjoy the journey

Jessica's Feedback

I have really enjoyed the flexibility of this program. Flexibility represents the freedom that you talked about. I love the freedom of choosing and feel pride with accomplishment. I am appreciative that these lessons are impacting not only my physical well-being, but my entire life experience.

Day 24

1. Alignment

2. Action: TT, Hamstring Stretch, Shoulder Rolls/Swimmers, Miracle Knee

3. Appreciation

Today, we're gonna start to learn about getting up from a chair or toilet with some ease. As you get stronger, getting up gets easier. Eventually, getting up turns into a great strength and stamina building exercise, which we call the Get Up.

On the way to the Get Up, we're gonna take the next couple days and approach the Get Up one small step at a time. No surprise there. TT is one of the best exercises to support your ability to get up from where you are sitting. Here's why: the heel-butt connection gives you access to firing your butt muscles as you begin to get up. Those muscles are the primary mover as you initiate getting up. Aren't you glad you've been practicing that?

TT heel butt initiates the Get Up, then Football Huddler takes over in the middle. Then you're up! I gave you instructions for the Football Huddler in the beginning of this chapter. In case you missed it, here's the abbreviated instructions:

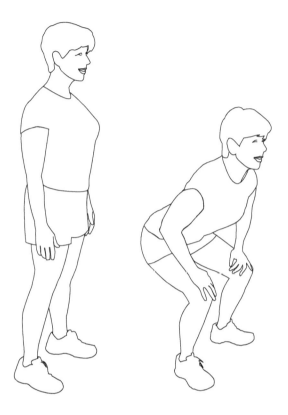

Football Huddler

Here's how you do the Football Huddler:

- Stand with your feet spread pretty wide.

- Bend your knees a bit as you put your hands on your thighs.

- Lean forward slightly as you stick your butt out a little.

- Keep your eyes forward.

- Imagine how the players look in a football huddle.

- You can hold it for a few seconds, then squeeze your butt as you come back to upright.

The next time you go to get up from a chair, initiate the get up with a TT heel dig and butt squeeze. Notice on your way to standing up, you pass through the Football Huddler position. As a matter of fact, why not try it right now? Sit on the edge of your chair, feet spread, and hands on thighs if you can reach. Rock forward, heel-butt connection, push off your thighs, Football Huddle position to standing upright. We'll be working on this together over the next couple of days and how you are with a Get Up will be evolving. Remember, you never get it done so you can't get it wrong.

Relax, I'm gonna give you lots of ways to make this manageable as we go along.

Jessica's Feedback

I am looking forward to practicing alignment with the Get Up. When I did it in the past, it was mentally forced. Admittedly, I currently dread getting into a standing position almost every time I stand.

Day 25

1. Alignment
2. Action: TT, Hamstring Stretch, Shoulder Rolls/Swimmers, Miracle Knee
3. Appreciation

More on the Get Up.

The Get Up excites me because it's a move that everyone needs to be able to do. At the same time making it more and more doable means it becomes a great way to build stamina. Getting up from a chair uses many large muscles—leg, thigh, and core—which means it requires a pretty big effort. More muscles recruited, more effort required. This required effort means that as getting up gets easier, you are getting stronger and building stamina—stamina to move around in the world. The Get Up is a great strength and stamina building exercise!

Start where you're at. No shame. No blame. Locate yourself on this continuum:

1. I cannot get up from a chair.
2. I can get up once with help and great effort.
3. I can get up but it ain't pretty.
4. I can get up.
5. I can get up with ease.

The Get Up

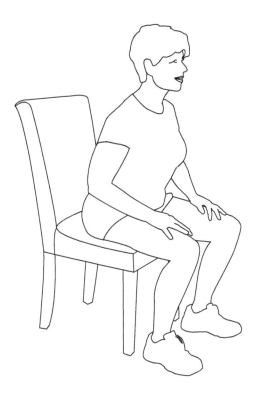

The Get Up

For everyone, here's the posture and procedure of the Get Up. Positioning yourself and using intentional muscle recruitment into a Get Up can make them instantly easier. You can use the exercises you've been doing in a specific way to do this.

- Sit as if you are ready to get up.

- Spread your legs a bit, wide but not too wide.

- Put your hands on your thighs if you can.

- To initiate the get up, rock forward slightly as you push out of your heels; squeeze your butt and push off your thighs with your hands.

- You are looking to get up into the Football Huddler position on route to standing up.

- To sit back down, go the Football Huddler and keep going lower until your butt hits the chair.

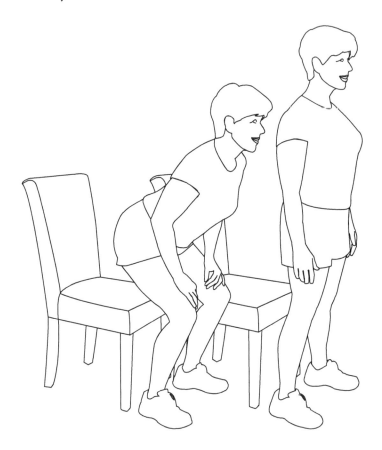

The Get Up

Often, this way of getting up makes it easier for many folks right away.

It's also empowering because the results of your TT will be used right here! Although this works for many, many people, bodies are very individual. If you have a way of getting up that is working just fine for you, then use that. I always give what has worked best for most of my people over the years, but there are always exceptions. Nothing's wrong, just all bodies are different. Some things work for most people. Everything never works for everybody.

Did you try a Get Up with the procedure I outlined? Did it become easier? Notice if this Get Up posture/procedure changes where you are on the continuum. Sometimes, your number will change. Today, as you move through your day. Notice how you are getting up. Use your butt muscles and your heel-butt connection intentionally. We call this intentional muscle recruitment (IMR). Notice the Football Huddler. Tomorrow, more on this getting up thing.

Here's to standing strong and moving forward!

Jessica's Feedback

Interestingly, the butt squeezes started helping me early on in my exercise path. They are especially helpful when my energy is low as it gives me that oomph from using those big muscles. I identify with number two and number three on the continuum scale. I am mostly able to "get up but it ain't pretty," (thanks for the very real humor). There are occasions where I will enlist help after sitting in lower seats or sitting for a long period of time. I have been using the "rocking" method to stand up for years. It takes a lot of momentum as you mentioned to get into a standing position.

I'm feeling anticipation and dread in adding Get Ups to my core exercises. The dread is mental. I feel it whenever I consider standing up and moving anywhere. Right now, the only thing that moves dread is accomplishing the physical task. Right now, sitting back down is the motivation to move anywhere. This habit, this alignment has been way off for a long time. Like I mentioned in yesterday's writing, I am looking forward to using the AAA practice when doing the Get Up. This is a really big deal in getting me mobile.

Day 26

1. Alignment

2. Action: TT, Hamstring, Shoulder Roll/Swimmer, Miracle Knee

3. Appreciation

Today, we're gonna go a little deeper into the Get Up. What did you notice yesterday about getting up? I forgot to mention yesterday that you can use AAA to smooth your Get Up path. Did you use intentional muscle recruitment (IMR) with your TT heel-butt connection? Did you notice the Football Huddler? Appreciate yourself for these days that you have been strengthening (TT and Miracle Knees) because it's been contributing to your Get Up success!

We're also gonna add the Heel Tap into your routine. Review the Heel Tap at the beginning of chapter 4 or find abbreviated instructions at the bottom of this page.

Locate yourself again on the continuum, in case it feels different today than it did yesterday (I fluctuate between three, four, and five).

1. I cannot get up from a chair.

2. I can get up once with help and great effort.

3. I can get up but it ain't pretty.

4. I can get up.

5. I can get up with ease.

The point is to be where you are and take it from there. No shame. No blame. Funny, that kind of sums up my whole book.

The only way to make Get Ups into a great strengthening and stamina creating exercise is to make it feel friendly. If you are at number one, number two, or number three, get a higher chair! A bar stool, a handicap toilet, or shower seat could work. You can put books, pillows, or some kind of box or block on your chair. Whatever you can do to make your chair higher, it makes it easier to get out of. As you get stronger, you can move to lower seats. We use the higher chair to make this a great strengthening exercise. Eventually, it will get easier to get up from lower places.

This is *not* about fighting your way up repeatedly from a seat that is hard for you to get out of. Get a higher chair. As many times as I say this, there are always folks who don't believe me. They keep struggling to get out of the chair. This is not what we're aiming for. Get a higher chair for the purpose of getting stronger. Make peace with where you are. The object is to get to number four and then begin to add repetitions, which will take you to number five. Remember, you never get it done so you can't get it wrong. Nothing behind, everything in front.

If you are at number one: Try from the highest chair you can find or create. Keep doing TT and Miracle Knee and add in the Heel Tap (Instructions at the end of this page). The object is to move to number two. Take your time, no hurry or pressure. Make peace with where you are.

If you are at number two: Move to a higher chair. See if that moves you up the scale. Keep doing TT and Miracle Knee. Add in the Heel Tap.

If you are at number three: Move to a higher chair and pretty that up; TT, Miracle Knees, and Heel Taps.

If you are at number four: Try doing a few in a row. Maybe two or three. When that feels easy, add another one. Keep doing all other exercises. You are welcome to do Heel Taps too.

If you are at number five: When a set of fifteen is easy, get a lower chair.

Heel Tap with a Tiny Tilt:

1. Sit in ninety-degree rule with upright posture

2. Do a small pelvic tilt and hold it gently

3. Straighten your right leg tapping your heel

4. Return to start position, relaxing the pelvic tilt

5. Repeat on the other leg

All the benefits of the Heel Tap will help make your muscles more able to get you up from a chair! Heel Taps are a great pre-Get Up move too.

Bonus: Doing a few Heel Taps before you get up from a sitting position helps relieve the stiffness that comes from sitting and makes getting up easier.

Jessica's Feedback

I appreciate the Get Up modification because lower seats take so much more effort for me to get to a standing position. The TT has been the most noticeable and effective tool that I use every time I stand. I feel IMR each time especially by planting my heels firmly on the ground and using them as the primary source in standing up.

Day 27

1. Alignment

2. Action: TT, Hamstrings, Shoulder Rolls/Swimmers, Miracle Knees, Heel Taps/Get Ups

3. Appreciation

Two viewing points on Get Ups:

Number one. Doing a Get Up in your exercise practice.

When you are adding Get Ups to your exercise practice, they must feel friendly. Easy in fact, so you can do a couple or a few. Yesterday, I gave you suggestions for making Get Ups feel friendly. Over time, you will notice a progression of getting stronger and being able to lower your Get Up seat height or add more repetitions.

If Get Ups, as an exercise, are not for you yet, then continue your exercise practice. You will get stronger. You will eventually find your way to a friendly feeling Get Up.

Below I will give you some options for adding Get Ups and/or Heel Taps to your exercise practice.

Number two. Getting up from where you're sitting.

If getting out of your seat is some degree of challenging, throw everything we've learned at it.

- AAA! Before you get up
- Use your heel-butt connection to intentionally recruit your butt muscles (IMR)
- Rock forward
- Push off your thighs or the arms of the chair
- Be curious about when you will notice it getting easier

- Look for signs that it's getting easier

- Keep your attention on what feels good about getting stronger

Practice options:

AAA TT, Hamstrings, Shoulders/Swimmers, Miracle Knee, Heel Taps (start with five on each leg and build from there).

AAA TT, Hamstrings, Shoulders/Swimmers, Miracle Knee, Heel Taps, Get Ups (friendly feeling, start with two or three and build from there).

Other options for Get Up strength building:

- Always use IMR when you are getting up.

- If the get up you just did felt good, try another one for the fun of it!

- If get ups are normally challenging and you find yourself on a bar stool or high chair, enjoy the ease and possibly do a couple, just for fun.

- I have a client who every time she pees, she does an extra get up.

- Be creative!

See you tomorrow!

Jessica's Feedback

Because you introduced Get Ups toward the end of the thirty days, I feel much more solid in my routine, which allows for ease and alignment versus dread; in addition, I am mindful every time I stand, paying attention to AAA and IMR. I added five more reps to Swimmers, Shoulder Rolls, and TT and added ten more seconds to Hamstrings (a favorite stretch, gets my sciatica every time), I really feel the difference.

Day 28

Might this be a rest day for you?

Or

1. Alignment

2. Action: TT, Hamstrings, Shoulder Rolls/Swimmers, Miracle Knees, Heel Taps/Get Ups

3. Appreciation

We spent a lot of time on the Get Up because getting up is something you need to do for the foreseeable future. The Get Up uses a lot of the strength you have been building, and it's nice to know that as you get stronger, getting up gets easier.

The Get Up makes it really important for you to work the Easy Fitness systems. Begin where you are then find the smallest, friendliest feeling next step. Moment to moment, what's true and what's next.

Use the three keys when you are challenging yourself.

1. Nothing behind, everything in front; keep your attention on what feels good about where you are going.

2. Don't give a damn about what anyone else thinks; keep your plans to yourself until they feel stable.

3. You can't get it wrong 'cause you never get it done; there's no hurry, all is well. Relax, enjoy the journey. Make peace with where you are and take it from there.

You always want to follow the ideas and inspirations that come when you are in alignment. Remember, voice of wisdom will feel calm and friendly, even when you are dealing with Get Ups.

Tomorrow will be review and the next day, we'll look at moving ahead. Breathe. Relax. You're doing just fine. You've got this.

Next Steps

Well, we're at the end of this book. If you are still reading, I suspect you are still exercising! Yahoo you!

"Next Steps Review" will be on Day 29 and includes a complete review including concepts and exercises.

"Next Steps Moving Ahead" will be on Day 30 and includes ideas for moving ahead on your own or getting more support.

Day 29
Review

Twenty-nine days in a row! Yahoo You! Yahoo me for writing this book!

1. Alignment

2. Action: TT, Hamstrings, Shoulder Rolls/Swimmers, Miracle Knees, Heel Taps/Get Ups

3. Appreciation

Concept Review

Easy Fitness is a system—a system that is friendly feeling and doable. A system that is easily repeatable. To work the system, you listen to your body. That's how you know what to do next. If you don't know exactly, then you try something small and friendly and see how it goes. No big deal. We practiced starting and stopping exercise during our time together so you have the skill to begin and begin again.

The system starts with AAA, which stands for Alignment+Action+Appreciation. Alignment is you being in a purposeful momentary good mood before you take action. Action is an Easy Fitness friendly feeling small step exercise and always comes after alignment. Appreciation is you feeling good about yourself for taking that small step. *The AAA system inspires your positive momentum making accountability and motivation obsolete.*

Alignment and appreciation (AAA) are wonderful neighbors, and it's fun and easy to move between them. Voice of wisdom lives in the same neighborhood as alignment and appreciation, and you can always hear it there. Voice of wisdom gives you access to listening and hearing what your body needs/wants next. Alignment, appreciation, and listening to your voice of wisdom put you in the stream of well-being, and there is no better place to be.

Three Easy Fitness keys that help you tap into your own wisdom and find your own path to improved strength and stamina, they are:

1. Nothing behind, everything in front. *Easy Fitness is a fresh start.*

2. Don't give a damn about what anyone else thinks. *Keep this to yourself until you feel steady at it*

3. You never get it done, so you can't get it wrong. *Relax, all is well. There's always another shot at it later or tomorrow.*

The Easy Fitness success formula: Doing what I said I would do about exercise consistently and without struggle.

Personal freedom and empowerment are inherent in this formula. Freedom and empowerment come from *you* saying what you will do and *you* having the capacity to follow through. The three keys help you stay on track with the Easy Fitness success formula. Keys 1 and 2 help you decide what's right for you to do, then do it consistently. Key 3 helps take the struggle out.

You learned that struggle can happen when you are doing nothing. Struggle is usually in your mind and comes from your thoughts. All our tools and systems help to minimize struggle, creating more ease for you on your path. When all else fails and struggle has a hold on you, take a nap.

The Easy Fitness Make a Choice Formula: What would a person who is willing to be happy and healthy do today?

1. Ask the question

2. Answer the question

3. Do the answer

Use this formula when you are not sure what your next step is. The answer should feel friendly.

Exercise Review

Tush Tilts, chapter 1

Hamstring/calf stretch, chapter 2

Shoulder Rolls, chapter 2

Swimmers, chapter 2

Miracle Knee, Chapter 3

Heel Taps, Chapter 4

Football Huddler, Chapter 4

Get Ups, Chapter 4

The concepts and exercises probably feel familiar to you. You've got this. You can use these exercises indefinitely. In the next section, we'll review how to increase, how to find new exercises, and how to get more support from me.

Jessica's Feedback

I have been at ease over the last four or five days, not freaking out if my AAA time passes or I do individual exercises at separate times. It doesn't feel like there's a whole lot of room for monkey mind on Day 29. I feel successful and strong. Get Ups are hard no doubt. So at this point, I am doing one structured Get Up a day; I practice IMR and AAA each time I prepare to stand. So I feel the task at hand now is to consistently change my thinking about getting up. Paying attention to my alignment when opportunities and/or the need to stand arises. As I wrote this, I felt monkey mind starting to create goals too big for where I am currently at. I stopped and will resource this goal regularly.

Day 30

Moving Ahead

1. Alignment

2. Action: TT, Hamstrings, Shoulder Rolls/Swimmers, Miracle Knees, Heel Taps/Get Ups

3. Appreciation

Here we are!

This is the end of the book but the beginning of your Easy Fitness life!

I suggest that AAA, TT be your "get back on track" routine if you ever need it.

Getting back on track is when you've slipped away from your practice and you want to restart. Relax, it's normal to get sidetracked or sidelined. Just take a breath, AAA TT and proceed from there. Sometimes, you can jump right back in. Sometimes, you build back up. Depends on how you feel.

Note the difference between coming back from a rest day and getting back on track.

How to Move Forward

Review of relaxed expansion guidelines: Knowing how to increase your exercising safely and successfully.

Are you ready to increase? Yes, if what you're doing feels easy and doable on a regular basis. If you feel relaxed and maybe even happy when you think about your current exercise promise, then it's time to think about how to add on.

Here are some terms that will help you:

- Repetitions or Reps. The number of times you do the actual movement

- Sets. A group of reps with a rest in between

- Frequency. How often

- Intensity. The actual amount of effort or circumstances that effect effort

- Duration. The length of time

Here are some guidelines:

- Reps: Increase reps, add one or two at a time

- Sets: Add a second set. When adding a second set, you can do less reps and work up to two sets of ten

- Frequency. Do your second set at another time

- Intensity: You can squeeze harder or add reps or decrease rest

- Duration: Add your second set at the same time, and you increase length of time exercising

There are a million different combos of the above. After you think it through, try it and see how it feels. If it feels doable but not quite as easy you're on the right track, you might try different combos to see what's best for you. For instance, if your mornings are crowded, you might want to do a second set of everything or something later in the day. Figuring this out and knowing how flexible you can be about it will give you freedom— freedom to choose what's exactly right for you!

How to find your next appropriate small step:

1. Follow me on YouTube to get some nifty small step exercise options.

2. If you like to dance, add a minute of chair or kitchen dancing. Just put on your favorite song and move around some. Really, start with thirty seconds or one minute and go from there. You can also do a search for chair dancing and follow a video. Start small!!

3. If you love to walk, pick an appropriate starting point and add a little bit each day. To find your starting point, figure out what is your current comfortable walking distance. I've had clients start at ten steps, one lap around the car, or a half block or more. Find your current comfortable walking distance, begin there and add approximately 10 percent at a time. When you are comfortable with the increase, then increase again. You will play this by ear, increasing in a way that is just right for you. A walking program might kick up all the "shoulds." Remember the keys!

4. Try a Google search for chair exercise or some other criteria and see what comes up. For instance, search for a calf stretch and see what comes. If something strikes your fancy, give it a try. Keep in mind that most options will have to be broken down into bitesize pieces. Small! Small! Small! And friendly too!

5. Schedule an Easy Fitness training session with me on the phone and together, we'll figure out your personal plan. E-mail coach@cinderernst.com or call 415-699-5797

6. Sign up for one of my coaching programs if you need more ongoing support, find out more at http://cinderernst.com

7. Check our website to attend an Easy Fitness workshop near you http://easyfitnessbook.com.

The Easy Fitness Way

Stay on board the Easy Fitness train. Remember, we built this foundation so you would have a way to proceed outside traditional fitness guidelines. Stay outside of traditional fitness guidelines. Trust yourself. Listen for your voice of wisdom. If it feels good, friendly and energizing, you're on the right track. Your feelings will tell you. Follow your emotional guidance system!

Have fun with this.

All is well!

You're doing just fine!